YOUR DOLLAR$, YOUR HEALTH:

HEALING STRATEGIES AND SKILLS

by

Roger G. Swartz, M.A.Ed., M.P.A.

and

Gretchen Peske, R.N., M.S.N.

with

Karen Pennebaker, B.A.

Published by Blue Path Press, Hockessin, DE
Printed by Wickersham Printing Company, Inc.,
Lancaster, PA
1996

First Edition

ISBN: 1-887109-00-5

Library of Congress Number: 95-76320

Cover design by Karen Pennebaker
Published by Blue Path Press, Hockessin, DE
Printed in the United States of America

For information on wholesale/quantity pricing or direct mail orders,
Telephone: 717-299-5061; FAX: 717-560-0522; e mail PAPenne@aol.com

This book was typeset in LotusWorks on a Packard Bell Legend 130CD Supreme,
Drawings scanned into Micrografx Picture Publisher with Mustek 6000CX.
Proofs printed on Hewlett Packard LaserJet IIP plus.
Body copy in 12 point Times New Roman.

TOPICAL TABLE OF CONTENTS

DEDICATIONS

I dedicate my work in this manuscript to my spouse, for continuing to practice preventive, comprehensive family medicine and for his constant support, patience and reassurance. Thank you, Derek!

- Gretchen Peske

To Lucia, for using the knowledge and skills of this book immediately following the automobile accident.

To those healthcare professionals advancing the field of patient education; and to those patients functioning in the role of co-therapist.

- Roger Swartz

ACKNOWLEDGEMENTS

The authors wish to express their gratitude to diverse people who have helped in the preparation of this manuscript. These include: Ellen Shenk and Stephen Mitchell, for editing; and Lucia Pollock, for proofreading.

A special thanks goes to Karen Pennebaker, who not only provided illustrations and a cover design for this book, but also prepared the book for printing; contributed suggestions on wording, compiled and provided the listing of alternative therapies and the internet resources; served as a viable link between the authors; and provided patience, perseverance and positive thinking throughout the last four years.

A special thank you to Melissa Jaquette, for providing typing services for Gretchen Peske.

Finally, the authors wish to express their gratitude to the organizations listed in the "Resources" section (Section #31) for taking time to provide descriptions of their services.

OVERVIEW

This book is primarily intended for healthcare professionals who have responsibility for patient education. These professionals come from many disciplines and their responsibilities span the continuity of care spectrum: from preventive medicine and wellness programming through hospitalization and discharge.

This book is also intended for the healthcare consumer who experiences health-related problems and uses services provided by the healthcare system. For the consumer, this book addresses such questions as:

- How do you talk with your doctor? What questions should you be asking about your prescribed treatment(s) and medications?
- How do you counteract the negative consequences of stress that always accompany a disease?
- What questions should you be asking in terms of joining a support group? How do you choose a group?
- What can you do to reduce your own out-of-pocket expenditures for healthcare services?

We, the authors, advocate patient education as a bridge leading to wellness. As such, the role of patient education is expanded into three major themes:

- Multidimensional healthcare strategies that incorporate the emotions and spiritual beliefs into the healing process
- Mind/body behavioral medicine interventions skills (see Section #18) incorporated into patient education, training, and teaching methods; and training the patient in ways to use such skills to facilitate healing
- Involvement of the patient as co-manager and co-therapist

For both the lay person and the professional, the overriding theme of healing and its four levels weave these three themes together. The healing stream and its levels nourish the strategies and skills presented, bringing them to life. As we present in this book, we believe that healing is "proactive wellness" rather than simply "reactive disease care." We do not have a healthcare system in this country. We do have several "disease care" components. (A system implies all component parts mutually supporting one another in an effective and efficient manner.)

In developing these themes, in describing the strategies and skills inherent within them, the authors present numerous resources and research documentations within the field of healthcare. And we offer mind/body behavioral interventions and related education and training skills as a *supplement* to prescribed treatment, *not* as a substitute for such treatment.

The book is designed for easy use by professionals and lay persons. The topical table of contents will help cross-reference the material quickly. A listing of reference numbers at the end of each section corresponds to the numbered sources in the Bibliography. Other relevant sections are cross-referenced within each section. To further aid the reader, Section #31 contains resources mentioned in some of the sections. Each section is broken down into subheadings, with bulleted information to highlight material. Hence, this book is constructed and written in order to serve as an easily accessed reference book.

The pre-publication notes update the state of this nation's healthcare crisis in terms of current trends to reform the healthcare system and curtail costs. In light of these trends, the need for patient education becomes more urgent.

Roger G. Swartz
Gretchen Peske
July, 1996

PRE-PUBLICATION NOTES

In the rapidly changing world of healthcare, it is difficult for a book to keep abreast of changes, especially those taking place in the private sector. This work is no exception; buthis section is an attempt to bridge the gap. The greatest change taking place today within the system is that of managed care. This section is an effort to characterize this concept and to detect its emerging advantages and disadvantages.
(Resources located at the end of this section have not been included in the main Bibliography.)

Managed Care

Managed care evolved from pressure by employers on insurance carriers to find lower cost alternatives to fund healthcare benefit packages for their employees as healthcare costs continue to escalate. Insurers began competing against each other to also control excessive use of high cost medical care in both private and public sectors. They did this by providing new methods of healthcare delivery intended to limit individuals and organizations from over-consuming and providers from both over-supplying benefits and mismanaging funds. At the present time, consumers are facing a wide variety of benefit options.

The term managed care refers to these innovations in the delivery and financing of healthcare services in the most cost effective manner possible. [NERA, 95]
The following trends have developed: [NERA, 33]

- Prospective reimbursement
- Influence of patients' choice of service providers
- Negotiation of payment terms with service providers
- Utilization controls and review management, in which any of the following can be done:
    - Establishment of acceptable norms for physicians
    - Review of hospital physician practices and discharge planning
    - Use of primary care physicians before referral is made to specialist

Manifestations of managed care are acronyms that are becoming household words: HMOs and, less common, PPOs. HMO stands for Health Maintenance Organization; PPO, for Preferred Provider Organization. Though the differences between these two are becoming less and less distinct, one major difference remains: within a PPO, the patient has greater personal choice as to primary caregiver.

Diagnostic Related Groups (DRGs) (Section #2) and prospective reimbursement have changed hospital profit incentives. In 1983, the year DRGs were instituted as a policy within Medicare, Medicare paid for 27.5 percent of hospital cost. [NERA, 38] Subsequent hospital managerial actions to continue profit included:

- Shorter hospital stays and more rapid patient discharge (covered in this text)
- Greater reliance upon out-patient surgery. [NERA, 23] By 1990, this accounted for 50 percent of all surgery performed. [NERA, 32]

This, in turn, resulted in these current developments: [NERA, 23]

- Increase in empty hospital beds/falling hospital occupancy rate
- Competition among hospitals for physicians and healthcare specialists as well as patients, as a result of falling occupancy rates

A contributing factor to this trend was the ability to obtain the necessary financial resources. [NERA, 23]

The Merger Movement

The above developments have led to the merger movement within managed care: this means, essentially, managed competition. In 1994, approximately 700 U.S. hospitals joined forces administratively, [Fried, PI, E1] in innumerable combinations, for the purpose of: [Fried, PI, E9]

- Cost reduction
- Efficiency in delivery of services. Various services can be provided under one administrative roof and the patients entered in one data base
- Patient care. Mergers allow studies of what practices or treatment works best, and quick dissemination of these findings to their staff

Mergers do have their critics. The primary criticisms are these:

- *What* cost reduction?
- *What* efficiency in delivery of services?

How many states have established administrative mechanisms to monitor medical costs and prices as a result of mergers within their political jurisdictions? Indeed, even those studies undertaken within the hospital industry itself, where research has been conducted, have found no direct correlation between lower costs and mergers. [Fried, PI, E9]

Mergers may actually increase healthcare costs. Citing one major industry-wide study, Fried stated that costs escalated because the larger institutions created by merger were still adding services after the merger was completed. [Fried, PI, E9] Thus, competition is but carried to a higher level, as one institutionally merged conglomerate is threatened by the competition potential of another conglomerate.

Fried also cites findings of a Senate committee for the state of Massachusetts which indicate that mergers can adversely affect delivery of services. [Fried, PI, E9] A facility, the committee found, can cut back on services and/or staff due to the financial pressures associated with merger.

Furthermore, the cost cutting pressures due to competition have the greatest effect on the weaker step-child of the merger (most often an inner city hospital) and is the one experiencing the cutbacks. This was the finding of an American Hospital Association study of hospitals that closed between 1983 and 1988. [Fried, PI, E9]

Managed Care or Managed Profit

The advantages of managed care have been listed above. However, managed care also has its criticisms. These are: [NERA, 91-129;130]

- Cost reduction
- High administrative costs
- Care focus versus cost focus?

Cost reduction. Is there sustained cost reduction within the managed care movement? Until recently, HMO and PPO premium level increases matched closely premium level increases in traditional, private insurer fee-for-service policies. [NERA, 91] A 1988 study of utilization review as a cost control found that administrative tool has a one-time impact upon cost reduction. [NERA, 90] A 1992 US Congressional Budget Office study concluded that utilization review procedures consisting of pre-certification and concurrent review of in-patient cases might reduce national healthcare expenditures by one percent. [NERA, 90]

High administrative costs. A 1995 CBS series of investigative reports on HMOs found that Chief Executive Officers of HMOs are paid approximately twice as much as a CEO of a similarly sized company [Arnot, CBS, 10]. Greiner states that administrative overhead costs in the United States account for nearly 20 percent of all healthcare costs, as compared to 4 percent in Canada. [EPI, 15] She also cites figures revealing the growing prominence of management in the United States. In 1968, there were 100 managers for every 1,260 nurses and 340 physicians. By 1992, the ratio had been reduced to 100 managers for every 370 nurses and 80 physicians. [EPI, 15]

Greiner also cites a study that reveals that the U S health system, with 1500 different insurance companies, employs 85% more managers than the publicly financed Canadian system. In another study comparing healthcare costs of 17 industrialized countries, the United States ranked sixteenth in total expenditure on nursing as a percentage of Gross Domestic Product. Only Turkey spent less. [EPI, 15] These research studies seem to indicate that a disproportionate amount of healthcare cost is consumed by administration.

Administrative cuts include all costs incurred in providing healthcare insurance that are not directly related to the delivery of healthcare services to the patient, such as staff salary costs. However, there are some hidden costs such as patient time costs, productivity losses, and staff costs. At what point does a nurse "go" to patient billing activity (administrative duties) from providing direct patient care as he/she is documenting medical records? Is not some of this time also administrative costs?

Furthermore, managed care has transformed the role of third-party payers from passive claims processors into very active participants in patient education and treatment. This necessitates staffing. And managed competition has also forced higher advertising and marketing costs as third party payers, managed care organizations, and merged healthcare conglomerates compete against one another.

Cost Focus Versus Care Focus. Managed care has given a new emphasis on the primary care physician as the initial gate keeper. However, in doing this, the movement has created a conflicting role for the doctor: She/he not only has to diagnose and prescribe treatment, but also to act as an agent for the managed care organization in keeping healthcare costs at a prescribed level. This removes the primary care physician yet another level from delivering services to the patient.

In the summer of 1995, a think tank, the Economic Policy Institute of Washington, DC, released a clinical research study on cost cutting and the quality of patient care encompassing six major hospitals and an HMO. The study's author, Ann Greiner, concluded that by decreasing the number of registered nurses in order to reduce costs (due to pressure from managed care companies to discount their prices) the hospitals studied implemented their Reductions in Force (RIFs) in downsizing their numbers of registered nurses with great care. However, she also concluded, the hospitals are still not certain about the effect of the RIFs on the clinical quality of care provided. [Connell, PI, A11; Greiner, EPI, 2-3]

Greiner also concludes that overall, regarding staff interviewed in all organizations studied, those interviewed indicate that clinical quality is adversely affected when staff-to-patient ratios are widened; when training is inadequate; and/or when overall staff skill competency is lessened [EPI, 40]. She also cites one study indicating that a lower RN percentage of nursing staff is a detriment to quality of care [EPI, 39].

The authors of this work would add this question: Is the patient also being further short changed on the quality of needed patient education?

The Need for Patient Education

Currently, efforts at healthcare reform, with or without any US government healthcare reform, are running in the direction of managed competition, mergers and managed care [NERA, 97], based upon the premise that the healthcare industry needs to be tightly monitored in order to stop the rate of ever increasing healthcare cost. [NERA, 57]

Considering these trends, and with hospitals discharging patients sooner in order to reduce costs, the need for patient education is more critical than ever. Not only must the patients themselves assume a greater responsibility for their own healing, but healthcare professionals must also provide skilled training for patients in how to assume this responsibility. This book addresses these needs.

Pre-publication Resources

Arnot, Dr. Bob, Health Correspondent, "HMOs, CBS Evening News with Dan Rather, July 24, 1995," transcript, pages 9-10.

Connell, C., "Reducing Number of Hospital Nurses to Cut Costs Gets Mixed Reactions," *Philadelphia Inquirer*, Sunday, July 30, 1995, A11.

Fried, John J., "The Jury is Still Out on Hospital Mergers," Business Section, *Philadelphia Inquirer*, Sunday, April 30, 1995, E1, E9.

Greiner, A., *"Cost and Quality Matters: Workplace Innovations in the Health Care Industry,"* (Economic Policy Institute: Washington, DC), 1995.

The Healthcare System in the United States: Financing Health Care with Particular Reference to Medicines, Vol. 14 (National Economic Research Associates: New York), 1993.

EVOLVING ROLES OF PATIENT EDUCATION

AND THE

HEALTHCARE PROVIDER

Notes

#1: PATIENT EDUCATION: BARRIERS AND OPPORTUNITY

Definition

Patient education is defined as planned, structured learning experiences using methodologies that impact both the patient's knowledge and life style behaviors as they relate to health (Ref. #4).

Historical Perspectives

The "formative era" for patient education in the United States encompassed the latter half of the 19th and early 20th centuries (Ref. #5). In the late 1800s, an awareness of tuberculosis (TB) as a leading cause of death began to emerge. The chronic nature of TB, its long-term duration and the requirement for patients to take medication over long periods of time, instilled an awareness that educational efforts would be needed to successfully combat it. Commensurate with this growing public awareness, the emerging interest in the welfare of children and mothers, as well as the reduction of infant mortality, led to the establishment in 1908 of the Division of Child Hygiene within the Health Department of New York City. In 1921, the U.S. Congress passed the Sheppard-Tower Act, providing for the establishment of prenatal and child health centers.

Health professionals engaged in a tug-of-war regarding education. With such technological advances as the stethoscope, the ophthalmoscope, and the laryngoscope, patients began to perceive doctors as competent based on skillful use of the instruments. Doctors allowed the instruments to more objectively remove themselves from focus on the total person to concentrate on the physical body. Studies revealed that doctors took literally the writings of Hippocrates, father of the Hippocratic Oath: telling the truth to a patient about severe illness was contrary to the patient's best interest. In addition, Hippocratic writings established the authoritarian nature of the doctor-patient relationship as well as the general uncommunicative nature of that relationship.

Spreading from Great Britain through the work of Florence Nightingale, a strong advocate that nurses should assume the role of patient teaching, visiting nursing was introduced in the United States in 1872. More nursing associations soon formed, with teaching as a major role. The decades 1890-1910 saw the establishment of schools of nursing; this further strengthened the involvement of the nursing profession in the educational role.

An interregnum occurred in patient education from the decades spanning 1930-1960, with little advancement in the field. The "contemporary period," (Ref. #5) which began in the decade of the 1960s, is still ongoing. (However, Bartlett [Ref. #5] believes the contemporary period ended in 1984 with the advent of prospective cost containment programming [Section #2].) Patient education is again visible and on the agenda due to social movements begun in the 1960s, such as:

- Civil rights
- Consumer awareness
- Self-help (such as preventive medicine)
- Women's rights and issues

The field is also visible due to the reasons in the subsection "The Emergence of Patient Education," which follows later in this section.

Characteristics of Patient Education

Patient education includes both the healthcare professional and the layperson as teacher/trainer and implies that the layperson must take an active role, becoming a co-therapist, or co-manager, in both the learning and healing processes. This mutual active participation is based upon certain assumptions and models of helping and coping.

In the *traditional medical model* (Ref. #93), the person facing/experiencing the health problem is not held responsible for the problem or for its solution. In this model, the healthcare practitioner assumes that the patients believe they are subject to diseases that are and shall be beyond their control. The patient needs expert diagnosis, prescription, and treatment to be able to accept his/her state of health, and then passively participate in its solution or failure. The advantage of this model is that it allows the person to obtain help without placing blame on him/herself for ill health or for failure of treatment. The disadvantage is that it fosters dependency. The patient is literally to be patient and the healthcare professional has the full responsibility for success or failure. This model is illustrated in A in Figure 1.1.

This definition of patient education is premised upon the *compensatory model of helping and coping* (Ref. # 93). In this model (B, Figure 1.1), patients are in need of specific expertise and services that can help them gain more control over their own lives. Healthcare staff mobilize the missing resources the patient needs by educating the patient to ask questions concerning the prescribed medical treatment. Where feasible, healthcare staff train the patient in the use of these resources, viewing the patient as a co-manager, capable of problem-solving and having more control in his/her life.

This model hastens growth. From this perspective, both the healthcare professional and the layperson are actively engaged in the process of patient education.

Within the compensatory model, the goals of patient education are (Ref. #93):

- Fostering self care which involves providing the layperson with more resources to manage his/her health and the transfer of care responsibilities formerly reserved for the healthcare system
- Informed consent, a legal doctrine: Has the patient consented to his/her care?
- Coping: cognitive, affective and psychomotor knowledge values and skills that enable an individual to minimize a threat (real or perceived)
- Compliance and adherence on the part of healthcare professionals to laws, rules and regulations regarding the implementation of patient education and its documentation

The disadvantage from the co-manager's perspective is that not everyone wants to assume greater control. From the healthcare system's perspective, not everyone wants to give up control.

Barriers to Patient Education

Redman (Ref. #93) has identified the following as barriers to effective patient education within the healthcare system itself:

- Lack of patient education materials and lack of a system (including resources) for keeping materials current
- Lack of time for such needed activity due to decreased length of stay and inadequate staff resources
- Lack of third party reimbursement for outpatient education that contributes to lack of resources because hospitals cannot bill for providing such services
- Lack of space for providing patient education services (see "Patient Education as Social Support," Section #24, and Section #10)
- Few teachable moments because of the physical condition as well as the stress and anxiety level of the patient

- Lack of time spent in preventive health education due to lack of resources and due to the main function of a hospital: crisis intervention
- Staff are not comfortable with the role of instructing patients or are not committed to the philosophy of transferring or sharing responsibilities for healing; the patient is viewed as falling under the traditional medical model

Additional barriers to patient education include the following:

- Patients may not want to assume greater responsibility for either preventive health or for greater control in the healing process
- They may have been taught to believe that the doctor is the authority and become conditioned to this belief
- They may be denying their disease
- They may be unable to afford the costs associated with traditional medicine and its concomitant services
- The technologies of modern medicine may contribute to this attitude: "I have health insurance. Let the machines take care of it."
- Patient education is an ever-emerging field. In our healthcare consulting and training experience, often patient education within an institution has no coordinating arm and unifying mission philosophy. The only exception to this may be in cases where an interdisciplinary committee implements programming and develops internal policy
- With no unifying arm having authority and responsibility, patient education becomes fragmented
- Considering lack of resources and compliance regulations, priority is given to documenting patient education activity, not assessing its effectiveness. Without knowing the effectiveness, a healthcare bureaucracy and/or third party payer is not likely to commit additional resources to patient education

The Emergence of Patient Education

Patient education, in spite of these barriers, is becoming a prominent factor in healthcare. Redman (Ref. #93) identifies the following emerging trends that are thrusting patient education into prominence:

(1) Preventive medicine. Now that the escalating cost of healthcare represents 14% or higher of gross domestic product, which represents over $900 billion, more and more emphasis has been placed on preventive care. The preventive care trend itself started in the 19th century.

(2) Increasing incidence of long-term diseases and disabilities. An increase

in the incidence of long-term diseases and disabilities (such as those associated with chronic pain) necessitates that the patient and the caregivers understand both the disease and the accompanying illness (See Section #5 for the distinction between disease and illness).

(3) Reduced hospital stays. Recent emphasis on cost containment within healthcare has led to reduced stays within hospitals. The previously expressed attitude, "let the machines take care of it," assumes skilled technicians operate the equipment. Now the equipment must be operated in the home by either the caregiver or the co-manager and this necessitates training.

(4) Medical ethics. In 1980, the American Medical Association approved a revised Principles of Medical Ethics. In this revision, a physician will make relevant information available to both the public and patients. Also, in 1980, the American Hospital Association approved the "Patient's Bill of Rights." (The full 12 steps contained in this document are listed in Ref. #93).

(5) The holistic health movement (Section #7). This movement fosters self-care and self-responsibility, treating the person as an integrated whole. Healing implies not only physical dimensions but also mental, emotional, and spiritual dimensions (Section #5).

(6) Legality. The Patient's Bill of Rights (Ref. #2) opens a hospital to legal action in the same way its personnel rules and regulations are held liable in civil action in a court of law. Various federal legislative acts also have reference to patient education. For example, the Omnibus Budget Reconciliation Act of 1990 (revised through 1993) provides that each state develop a drug use review program that includes 11standards (such as side effects) for pharmacists who are counseling consumers in the drugs prescribed by a doctor either at the point of sale or the point of distribution.

(7) Accreditation. The Joint Commission on Accreditation of Healthcare Organizations has adopted standards relevant to patient education. These, along with many other diverse standards spanning all disciplines, serve as accreditation criteria for a healthcare organization. Table 1.1 lists the Education of Patients and Family Standards that are relevant to patient education (Ref. #61).

(8) Healthcare cost containment. Patient education is effective in containing the costs of healthcare (Section #2).

(9) Effectiveness of behavioral training. The emergence of mind/body behavioral medicines within traditional medicine, their results, and their impact upon healthcare costs (Section #2) provide justification for patient educators and other healthcare professionals sharing responsibility for education and training to begin to train patients on their use. This trend is closely related to number (5), above.

(10) New learning methodologies. The application of mind/body

behavioral medicine interventions used for healing are also used as training methodologies, such as in the field of accelerated learning. Accelerated learning has been successfully applied to staff development. (Refs. #55 and #80) These learning methods can also be used in patient education (Section #10).

These trends necessitate a new paradigm, from the traditional medical model, as symbolized in A, Figure 1.1, to that in B, Figure 1.1, representing the compensatory model of helping and coping, with the patient functioning in an active role as co-therapist.

References: 2, 4, 5, 55, 61, 80, 93

Table 1.1: EDUCATION OF PATIENTS AND FAMILY*: STANDARDS OF THE JOINT COMMISSION ON ACCREDITATION OF HEALTHCARE ORGANIZATIONS

(*Family refers to the person(s) who plays a significant role in the patient's life. This includes an individual(s) who may or may not be legally related to the patient.)

PF.1. The patient's learning needs, abilities, preferences, and readiness to learn are assessed.

PF.1.1. The assessment considers cultural and religious practices, emotional barriers, desire and motivation to learn, physical and cognitive limitations, language barriers, and the financial implications of career choices.

PF.1.2. When called for by the age of the patient and the length of stay, the hospital assesses and provides for patients' academic education needs.

PF.1.3. Patients are educated about the safe and effective use of medication, according to law and their needs.

PF.1.4. Patients are educated about the safe and effective use of medical equipment.

PF.1.5. Patients are educated about potential drug-food interactions, and provided counseling on nutrition and modified diets.

PF.1.6. Patients are educated about rehabilitation techniques to help them adapt or function more independently in their environment.

PF.1.7. Patients are informed about access to additional resources in the community.

PF.1.8. Patients are informed about when and how to obtain any further treatment the patient may need.

PF.1.9. The hospital makes clear to patients and families what their responsibilities are regarding the patient's ongoing health care needs, and gives them the knowledge and skills they need to carry out their responsibilities.

PF.1.10. With due regard for privacy, the hospital teaches and helps patients maintain good standards for personal hygiene and grooming, including bathing, brushing teeth, caring for hair and nails and using the toilet.

PF.2. Patient education is interactive.

PF.3. When the hospital gives discharge instructions to the patient or family, it also provides these instructions to the organization or individual responsible for the patient's continuing care.

PF.4.1. The hospital identifies and provides the educational resources required to achieve its educational objectives.

PF.4.2. The patient and family educational process is collaborative and interdisciplinary, as appropriate to the plan of care.

Figure 1.1: MODELS OF HEALING

A. The Traditional Medical Model:

DOCTOR

Patient.................Other Healthcare Professionals

B. The Emerging Medical Model:

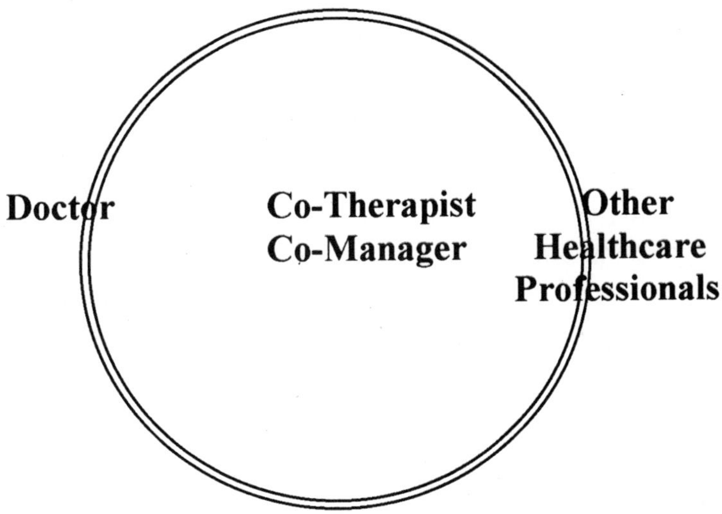

Key:

(solid line bracket) = lines of authority and responsibility, flowing from the doctor to the patient and other healthcare professionals

. . . . = line of communication, from healthcare professional to the patient

(double line) = shared lines of authority, responsibility and communication

#2: PATIENT EDUCATION AS COST CONTAINMENT

Background

Though patient education has been recognized as being integral to patient care in hospitals for the last few decades, only recently has the awareness developed that the function of patient education needs to be managed, as other components of patient care are managed. Management functions traditionally pertain to planning, coordinating, evaluation, fiscal accountability, and staffing. The need for management within the field has been brought about by such forces as:

- Increases in long-term chronic diseases and increases in the population having such diseases
- The need for documentation of the impact of patient education in coordinated, multidisciplinary treatment plans
- The implementation of such tools as the problem-oriented medical record
- The consumer, self-help movement with its demands for more information and greater responsibility in the individual's treatment
- Hospital administrative responsibilities related to informed consent, liability, and other legal matters
- Accreditation standards related to patient education (Ref. #93)

Fiscal forces have also provided major impetus for patient education to justify its impact upon treatment and cost containment. National expenditures for hospital care alone gained 61 percent from 1965 through 1980. This represented an increase of approximately $86 billion in those 15 years (Ref. #49). Currently, total healthcare costs represent approximately 14 percent or greater of the Gross Domestic Product, which equates to $900 billion or greater.

By the early 1980's, federal and state share of the bill for hospital care, due to enacted programs such as Medicare and Medicaid, was 54 percent (Ref. #49). Hence, since 1980 public policy related to healthcare has shifted to a focus of cost containment.

Both federal and state governments have designed various regulatory programs to curb healthcare cost. Three major types were initiated:

- Utilization controls, designed to minimize expenditures by prohibiting unnecessary days of care as well as inappropriate services
- Certificate-of-need requirements, restricting unnecessary capital outlays,

such as expensive equipment

- Budget/rate setting programs, either on a retrospective or prospective basis (Ref. #49)

Retrospective programs determine approved costs after the services are provided.
Prospective programs, such as the Diagnostic Related Groups (DRGs) establish reimbursement prior to the service.

In October 1983, the prospective payment system to hospitals based on DRGs was instituted. The federal government dramatically altered the nature of Medicare reimbursement to hospitals with the change from cost-based retrospective reimbursement to prospective payment. This reflected Congress' determination to curb ever-escalating Medicare program expense. The impact in terms of patient care was that hospitals would, in essence, be monetarily rewarded for discharging patients after shorter lengths of stay. Had the Medicare program continued to grow without restrictions, some, such as the Board of Trustees of the Social Security Program, feared funds for major components of Medicare would have been exhausted by the end of the 1990s (Ref. #54).

In addition to saving federal and state costs, other rationales behind DRG reimbursement programs were:

- The use of DRG data bases in community-wide collaborative planning
- The use of DRG data bases in quality assurance programs as an evaluation tool in evaluating medical care plans
- The encouragement of intra-hospital departmental coordination through encouraging physician, nursing, patient services and personnel to collaborate in providing quality care and expediting paper work (Ref. #49). (Also see "Allocation of Resources", Section #6)

Implications of Cost Containment

What impact does cost containment programming have on the patient, family and hospital system? These results occur:

(1) The healthcare provider becomes responsible for treating and discharging patients to return to the highest level of functional capacity in the shortest period of time.

(2) Current cost containment programming (see Preface) also creates the need for patients to obtain necessary skills and knowledge in home health treatment prior to discharge. Thus, the patient becomes a manager within the

healthcare system, a co-manager of both disease and illness (Section #5). This decreases the chances of hospital readmission. Readmissions are astronomically high for both hospitals and patients, not only in terms of money but also in terms of stress and anxiety. To circumvent hospitalizations, patients can be taught how to be pro-active health managers. This helps reduce costs. (See "Other Results...", below.)

The Patient Education/Cost Containment Research Data Base

A recurring problem for patient education is financing. A majority of insurance companies have not been willing to recognize patient education as reimbursable (Ref. #93). A critical component in obtaining reimbursement is in demonstrating its impact upon cost containment and healing. Major research findings on such impact are summarized as follows.

Lipetz, et al, (Ref. #68), state that patient education is in a "catch 22" situation. Very few patient education programs qualify for reimbursement. Furthermore, since such educational efforts are time consuming and compete with limited staff time for other tasks to be performed, it will not be seen as important as those other tasks or take precedence unless reimbursed in a specific budgetary category. Reimbursement by third party payers would bolster patient education programs within an institution as a higher priority task to be performed.

Redman (Ref. #93) cites numerous references demonstrating the efficacy of patient education upon healthcare. Particularly, note the three *meta-analyses* (research of the research) cited by Redman (Ref. #93) and Ornstein and Sobel (Ref. #81) that investigate the impact of patient education upon healthcare cost involving reduced stay. These three meta-analyses are References #32, #33 and #76. They collectively involve 185 research studies relevant to patient education, healthcare and cost.

The advantages of meta-analysis are:

- Trends that can be missing from one single isolated study can be identified with several studies
- Statistical methods employed are used to objectively quantify the overall data base. This eliminates subjectivity that may be involved in traditional methods of data collection by hand, one study at a time
- They also take into account overlapping content

Mumford, Schlesinger, and Glass reviewed 34 studies (Ref. #76). In their analysis, they discovered that:

- Patients in the experimental treatment group who were provided information and emotional support showed:
    - Cooperation with treatment
    - Increased speed of recovery
    - Fewer post-hospital complications than those patients in the control group who did not receive information or emotional support
- Ten of these 34 studies indicated that patients provided with information and social support had approximately, on the average, two fewer days in the hospital

Devine and Cook (Ref. #33) investigated, via meta-analysis, 49 studies, 9 of which were included in the Mumford, et al, study (above). Their key finding was that appropriate psychoeducational interventions reduce hospital stay by approximately one and 1/2 days. Such interventions included:

- Provision of information relevant to surgical procedures, pain, etc.
- Skills training (Section #10) relevant to post-operation exercises designed to: promote recovery, prevent complications, and reduce anxiety
- Psychosocial support given by the healthcare provider

Devine and Cook (Ref. #32) performed meta-analyses of 102 studies (44 of the studies appearing in Ref. #33 are incorporated into Ref. #32), to ascertain how psychoeducational interventions impact these four factors among adult surgery patients:

- Recovery (including length of hospital stay, medical complications, etc.)
- Pain
- Psychological well-being
- Satisfaction with care

Controlling for threats to internal and external validity, their findings were that statistically reliable effects were obtained for each of the four factors under consideration.

To understand the research findings, keep in mind that the effect size (ES) is a standard deviation score. Statistically, it is the average between the treatment and control group on the outcome variable divided by the standard deviation from the mean of the control group (Ref. #76). The ES signifies improvement (positive score) or loss (negative score) that any average member of a control group would experience if given the experimental treatment.

Devine and Cook's specific findings were as follows:

- Recovery: ES = +.50. A 95% confidence interval statistic for the sample of studies included in this factor, 73, ranges from +.41 to +.59. The ES is within this range. Thus the possibility of the results occurring by chance, only 5 percent, falls within the range of research acceptability. The positive ES score, +.50, signifies a positive difference in scores between the experimental/treatment group and the control group. Hence, the positive score favors the group receiving psychoeducational interventions

- Pain: ES = +.39. A 95% confidence interval for the sample of studies involved in this factor, 51, ranges from +.30 to +.48. Thus the ES is within this range. Here psychoeducational interventions reliably reduce surgical pain

- Psychological well-being: ES = +.40. A 95% confidence interval for the sample of studies included in this factor, 36, is +.22 to +.58. Psychoeducational interventions increase the psychological well-being of surgical patients

- Satisfaction: ES = +1.49. A 95% confidence interval for the sample of studies involved in this factor, 5, is +.23 to +2.74. The conclusion is that psychoeducational interventions increase the level of satisfaction surgical patients have with their care

What were the psychological interventions employed to obtain these results? They were essentially the following three types reported in the earlier Devine and Cook study (Ref. #33):

- Information involving:
    - Medical procedures
    - Needed life style behavioral changes
- Training skills, designed to:
    - Reduce discomfort
    - Promote recovery
- Psychosocial support designed to:
    - Reduce anxiety
    - Enhance self-coping

Other Results: How Patient Education Improves Healthcare

With increasingly shorter hospitalization stays, the demonstration that patient education can further reduce hospitalization time may be impractical. It is the proverbial squeezing blood from a turnip. However, researchers should begin to investigate whether such education and training helps reduce readmittance, thereby reducing cost. The Goldstein research article (Ref. #47) is an example of such investigation.

The Goldstein study is also interesting because it involves *training*, not just education, at a formal hospital-sponsored learning center for patients and caregivers. For a description of the learning center (Ref. #46), see Section #10, Table 10.1. For a discussion of patient education as social support, see "Patient Education as Social Support", Section #24, which includes the results obtained by this learning center.

In 1989, the International Patient Education Council (Section #31) published a Resource Sheet that listed the following eight major areas in which patient education was demonstrably shown to improve healthcare (Ref. #85).

(1) Patients adequately informed and prepared for surgical procedures:
- Encountered less pain
- Had less anxiety
- Developed fewer post-surgical complications
- Needed less time in the hospital

(2) Studies consistently showed that patient satisfaction improved when courtesy was displayed and patients received information.

(3) Patient adherence to the regimen of prescribed treatment was increased.

(4) Quality of life was increased.

(5) Patient control of chronic conditions (such as pain, asthma, chronic obstruction pulmonary disease, diabetes, and hypertension) was improved.

(6) Emergency room visits and hospital use were reduced. One study indicated diabetes-related hospital admissions were reduced by at least 50 percent.

(7) Health promotion efforts aided patients in disease prevention through life style behavioral modification.

(8) Mortality rates were decreased.

One of the main themes of this book is the integration of behavioral medicine into patient education, either as training methodologies (Section #10) and/or as healing mechanisms that the patient as co-therapist can be trained to use. For an example of the impact of behavioral medicine interventions upon cost containment, the reader is urged to consult Section #18, "Physical Benefits Derived from the Relaxation Response".

Other Considerations

Patient and behavioral medicine interventions work. As stated in the "Overview", this nation does not have a healthcare system but a disease treatment system. Furthermore, all of the components of the "system" have their own constituencies and interests.

Rarely will a hospital administrator (who have, as a group, a national mean cognitive processing style of 1-1-2-2; see Section #9 and Appendix B) increase the resources available for patient education for his/her institution; and/or reallocate already scarce resources to patient education and behavioral medicine endeavors, when they reap, as Devine and Cook state (Ref. #32), few benefits. Consider this line of reasoning: Why should my hospital put up the resources and bear the brunt of the cost? All the benefits accrue to the patient, the national interest, the government (for reducing medical costs), and/or the insurance companies, who do not reimburse for providing such services yet who benefit from healthier policy holders.

Patient education services exist in a "catch 22" situation. They must be performed and documented; accreditation bodies require it. However, without staffing and other adequate resources, there is no time for research. Without research results demonstrating its efficacy, third party payers will not reimburse for providing such services. Without reimbursement, administrators are reluctant to commit resources beyond what is needed to meet accreditation standards.

Policy makers in federal and state legislatures and executive branches need to enact legislation and promulgate rules and regulations that create incentives for healthcare organizations and third party payers to:

- Provide patient education services and/or reimburse for such services
- Engage in collaborative planning for service delivery with other healthcare providers within the community
- Provide funding for research and evaluation of different service delivery systems. (An agency such as the newly created Division of Alternative Medicine, National Institutes of Health [1993], becomes a vehicle for research, development and evaluation efforts)
- Shift emphasis from disease treatment and toward disease prevention. This includes the promotion of fiscal incentives for healthcare consumers

to adopt life style behaviors that foster prevention

Other questions must also be addressed in a total healthcare system that has as one of its cornerstones the policy of cost containment. Among these questions are:

- Should there be a place for euthanasia within cost containment? This would involve the elderly experiencing:
  - The latter stages of Alzheimer's Disease
  - Institutionalization due to mental illness combined with degenerative, incurable physical disease. (This might also pertain to those severely deformed at birth with no hope of recuperation)

- Should there be a place for rationing the healthcare dollar? At what point do multiple organ transplants become cost prohibitive when research indicates that within a few years, rejection of those organs occurs? At what point are cojoined twins not separated in order to possibly save one? At what point are victims of violence not treated, given their propensity and past criminal record for performing violent acts against society?

These are questions no longer confined to medical ethics or midnight coffee klatches. Cost containment, as a policy unto itself, and healthcare reform, as public policy involving cost containment, have thrown open the door for public policy debate on such matters.

References: 32, 33, 46, 47, 49, 54

#3: EMERGING ROLES OF THE HEALTHCARE PROVIDER

Continuity of Care

One result of the decreased time the patient spends in the acute care setting is the increased need for professionals in the healthcare arena to provide continuity of care following discharge. This need has been reinforced in healthcare association public policy statements, within accreditation body standards, and within governmental efforts of cost containment.

In 1972, the American Hospital Association included the following tenets pertaining to continuity of care within its adopted Patient's Bill of Rights (Refs. #2 and #93):

- Reasonable continuity of care is an inherent healthcare right of the patient
- Following discharge, the patient has the right to expect that the hospital will provide him/her logistical mechanisms for informing him/her of healthcare requirements

The 1994 Joint Commission on Accreditation of Healthcare Organizations (JCAHO) standards on evaluation of patient care state, in part, that discharge instructions must not only be given to the patient and/or the patient's family, but also to the organization responsible for continuity of care (Ref. # 61).

The government has mandated that patients spend fewer days in the hospital to cut costs as a result of the Diagnostic Related Groups' payment system instituted in 1983 (Section #2). Healthcare groups mandate patients be made aware of their healthcare needs prior to discharge. Consequently, the healthcare professional has been challenged to provide care in the hospital and continuity of care from the hospital to home.

Healthcare Profession Attitudes

The behavior of healthcare professionals directly impacts the health and wellness of patients. What healthcare professionals view as a health crisis might not be one at all in the eyes of the patient. The ability to respond to the healthcare needs of the patient is one major responsibility of the healthcare provider. So often in the healthcare profession, healthcare providers expect more of themselves than just responding to the needs of the patient. Nurses, in particular, will admit to experiencing guilt when there is not enough time to accomplish what the nurse thinks needs to be done.

Other questions healthcare professionals need to address include:

- Do nurses truly feel that they must "do it all"? And if so, when will nurses begin to ask for help from other disciplines to provide care for their patients?
- What characteristics presently project an "image" of a health care provider?
- Do healthcare professionals need to change their image to help the patient move towards becoming a partner in care?
- What might help healthcare professionals create the appropriate image?
- Does the term *health* differ from the term *wellness*? (Section #18)
- How does physical curing differ from health?
- What is the differentiation between the concepts of illness and disease? (Section #5)

At an October 1992 meeting with Anne Dixon, Associate Director, Standards Department, of the JCAHO in Chicago, Ms. Dixon and co-author Peske shared the following mutual concerns about the nursing profession:

- Nursing mentality needs to change from being *acute task oriented* to being more encompassing
- Preparation for nurses must encompass health education and preventive medicine as well as acute care
- The role of teacher in nursing preparation is vague and must be clarified
- Nurses are constantly teaching; but the instruction needs to be documented
- Nurses need to increase relationships with other disciplines
- Within patient education, nurses cannot do it all. Nurses must include other disciplines in collaborative planning, implementation and evaluation efforts

Given the fact that accreditation bodies and federal and state government are mandating that disciplines collaborate to provide quality care and contain costs (Ref. #61 and Section #2), how can that be accomplished if professionals in hospitals do not work together? Some hospital professionals view their jobs as necessary for economic security alone, experiencing little, if any, satisfaction. A philosophy which can easily pervade and destroy morale is: "Here today, gone tomorrow." Long term commitments of hospital employees to hospital administration and vice versa are waning.

Changes from a department focus to cross over of disciplines will provide higher quality of care in healthcare institutions. JCAHO will ask hospitals: What have you been doing? How have you been doing it? What effect does it have? Does it need to be changed? All employees of institutions will attend organizational orientation in addition to department orientation (This is concurrent with the multidisciplinary approach philosophy.) Crossing over and working with other disciplines will enhance working together within a particular organizational culture. Employees will not be required to become reoriented when changing departments. The gaps between departments will be minimized as all employees are working for the same institution within the same corporate culture.

Patient Education Within Continuity of Care

What is the role and responsibility of the healthcare provider? The authors believe that the healthcare provider must create the environment for self-motivation and healing to take place. The term *responsibility* (consisting of the words *respond* and *ability*) promotes a *pro-active* concept whereby the healthcare provider is not ignoring the needs of the patient, but responding to them. Is the healthcare provider using resources within the healthcare systems to adequately respond to the patient's needs?

Given a multidisciplinary approach to patient care, other disciplines need to cooperate with healthcare teaching. Documentation of interventions made becomes essential. If patient teaching is begun by the nurse and continued by the respiratory therapist, *continuity of documentation* must be visible. Clear, concise, easy-to-read documentation is critical. As an example of this, representatives from Medicare offices are now telling physicians "if we can't read it, we won't pay for it." Consequently, many more physicians are using dictating equipment in their offices than ever before.

In the institutional settings, it is critical that clear documentation accompany the patient from service to service, department to department, and discipline to discipline. This will provide a true multidisciplinary approach to caring for the patient and a good record of patient teaching which the individual receives.

Teaching the patient how to provide self-care skills at home to complete the sickness/wellness cycle becomes the responsibility of the healthcare provider.

Physical, mental, emotional, and/or social factors may create certain pitfalls when a person becomes a patient. Patients:

- Are prematurely discharged sicker and quicker
- Recuperate slowly
- Lack adequate at-home care providers
- Cannot perform self-care skills adequately
- Often receive poor discharge teaching/training from the hospital

What are other responsibilities of the healthcare provider with reference to patient education?

- Recognize personal/environmental limitations of time for bedside teaching
- Learn and practice effective communication skills
- Identify informal needs of patients
- Identify informational needs of patients
- Give patients the necessary skills and knowledge that foster the healing process
- Increase multidisciplinary cooperation and collaborative planning

The changes in healthcare that are forcing expanded roles of health educator upon all healthcare providers are resulting in a broad approach to the patient. The patient needs to be viewed as a part of a social system outside of the acute care setting. The objective of hospital care is to treat and discharge the patient as quickly and cost effectively as possible. How then will the healthcare provider focus on post-hospital care when the patient is in the hospital bed? Is the patient in the hospital bed ready to receive the information the healthcare provider wants to provide? The concept of *readiness to learn* is an important element in the patient education/teaching/learning cycle. Learning is a two way street. It is a process between at least two people in which there is fluidity with exchange of information. Committing to the process of patient education is the responsibility of the healthcare provider. By committing to the process, the healthcare provider can create the environment for learning. This, then, is the primary focus and the responsibility of the healthcare provider.

In the teaching relationship, the professional and/or caregiver is responsible for providing the learning environment. How to do this becomes a challenge as time is limited and comfort and energy are often nonexistent. What are the forces affecting the healthcare provider who is trying to provide teaching instruction to the patient? The healthcare provider attempts to do the job, constrained by the following forces:

- Lack of time

- Acutely ill patients
- Vague notion of the role of the teacher
- Overwhelming tasks
- Conflict of multidisciplines (Example: Whose job is it, really?)
- Inadequate staffing
- Lack of reimbursement
- Lack of understanding of how adults learn
- Nurse's compulsion to do a thorough job
- Patient's rejection
- Inadequate motivation on the part of the nurse and patient

Only when patient educators appreciate the barriers preventing them from teaching will the job really get done. Many hospitals are establishing patient education committees and appointing chair people of these committees to research and develop methods to teach the patient. The role of the patient education coordinator within continuity of care is threefold:

- Provide instructions to groups and individual patients
- Provide encouragement to clinical staff performing patient teaching duties
- Act as a resource for the staff to obtain materials for patient teaching

By crossing over the territorial lines of the multitude of disciplines in healthcare, by taking the risk to perform patient teaching actions, by encouraging the patient's family to actively participate and learn self-care skills, the healthcare provider is accepting responsibility with the patient to teach and enhance the self-care skills that will provide continuity of care.

References: 2, 61, 93

THE PATIENT AS PARTNER,

CO-MANAGER,

CO-THERAPIST

Notes

#4: EMERGING ROLES OF THE PATIENT

Overview

Our healthcare system is not a system at all. The meaning of the word *system* implies an organized whole consisting of component parts. Our present healthcare system has component parts in direct conflict and competition with one another.

Two major goals of this book are to identify knowledge and skills that the healthcare provider teaches the patient to perform and to identify the knowledge and skills needed by the patient to assume these roles.

Continuity of Care: From the Hospital to Home Health

The patient (a person experiencing disease and/or illness: Section #5) is directly affected by societal and economic pressures, even political pressure.

The change from retrospective reimbursement (reimbursing a hospital after patient discharge) to prospective payments (reimbursing a hospital prior to admission based on what a performed service should cost) reflected the United States Congress' determination to reduce Medicare expenditure. (See Section #2 regarding DRG's.) This prospective payment system meant also that hospitals would, in essence, be reimbursed for discharging patients after an average length of stay. This has decreased the number of recuperative days a patient spends in an institution. This has produced cost containment for hospitals and taxpayers by reducing Medicare expenditures.

This major policy decision within the healthcare system at best implies two major assumptions:
(1) Patients and families are physically able to care for the patient during the period of recuperation.
(2) This is accomplished in such a way that readmissions for the same problem are kept to a minimum.

Historically, prior to DRGs, the patient need not be concerned with developing responsibility for his/her self-care. This changed as of 1983. Redman, the Executive Director of the American Nurses Association, has stated that each patient now receiving treatment in our healthcare system has learning needs related to diagnosis, treatment, and prevention (Ref. #93).

These goals can only be achieved if the healthcare provider allows and encourages the patient to be an active participant in healthcare (Section #3). Patients must be given the opportunity to participate in their treatment as much as desired during their hospitalization, prior to discharge, if they are to continue the self-care process at home.

Patients must not only take advantage of any opportunity offered by healthcare providers, they must insist upon it, taking advantage of hospital accreditation standards relevant to patient and family education and patient's rights (Section #1).

Pertinent questions the patient (as co-therapist, partner, or co-manager) should be asking are as follows:

- What are the "payoffs" for my getting sick? (Examples: rest, built-in excuses for not being active, getting out of the "rat race", getting attention, etc.)
- Do I want to get well?
- Who really pays the bill? Does my insurance cover it? What percentage is left for me to cover?
- Do I understand the diagnosis?
- Do I understand the treatment?
- Do I have the skills, knowledge, and resources (including supplies and equipment) to continue treatment upon discharge?
- Do I understand the measures I can take following discharge to avoid readmission?

Policy directions are creating the need for a patient to play a more active role. There are other reasons:

- Mind/body therapies as outlined in this book (Section #18) do supplement traditional medicine

  For example, learning stress management skills can prepare you, the reader, for surgery and accelerate the healing process. Such skills can give you a greater sense of control, which is itself therapeutic ("Hardiness", Section #18)

- By becoming a co-therapist, you can improve communication with your doctor (Section #8). This can aid in your diagnosis and treatment and can foster a trust relationship with your doctor

References: 48, 49, 93

#5: INTEGRATION: THE FOUR LEVELS OF HEALTH

Healing: A Definition

The word *heal* is derived from *heilig* (German) and *hal* (Old English): holy and whole, respectively. Dr. Naomi Remen, medical director of Commonweal Cancer Help Program (Bolines, California), has described healing as "the movement toward wholeness" (Ref. #95).

The Four Levels of Health

Healing, or wholeness, has four components or levels:

- Physical
- Mental
- Emotional
- Spiritual

These components, which include matter, mind and spirit, are what make us human. They permeate Western science such as interdisciplinary systems theory and Western and Eastern psychologies and religions. (For a fuller discussion, refer to Refs. #42, #58, #92, #101, and #110. See also Table 5.1.)

Physical Health: Disease Emphasis

One major disadvantage of traditional medicine, many alternative medicine modalities and New Age therapies is their emphasis upon only one of the four components. Traditional medicine emphasizes the physical. Alternative, New Age therapies emphasize the spiritual (Section #7).

Consider this example: For the first time, Martha Thomas discovers a lump in her breast. Immediately, images of cancer spring to mind. She remembers her mother and aunt dying of metastasized breast cancer. The emotions of fear and helplessness grip her. She is not in control. She may even think, consciously or subconsciously, that God is punishing her.

This example indicates that illness is not disease. *Illness* is the subjective, emotional/mental experience of the disease and how the disease affects the patient's spirit. *Disease* is the physiological symptoms and/or biological damage visible (empirically proven) to a doctor. Doctors are trained to make a physiological diagnosis and prescribe treatment as soon as possible. This is the emphasis within *allopathic*, or Western medicine, which we now consider to be *traditional* medicine.

Failure to take into account the other components interacting with the physical disease may prolong and/or complicate treatment.

Mental Health Attributes

Mental health attributes include the use and application of all cognitive processing and learning styles (Section #9). This leads, in turn, to greater daily application of critical thinking skills involving linear thinking (logic and reasoning) as well as bilateral processing using both brain hemispheres. (See the listing of brain hemisphere functions in Section #9).

The acquisition of critical thinking skills also leads to increased problem-solving abilities. You, the reader, acquire greater skills in:

- Seeing how different elements of situations are related
- Having greater tolerance of ambiguous situations: rarely are things as black and white as they appear on the surface
- Possessing a greater Intelligence Quotient (IQ) in terms of not necessarily math and language abilities but in terms of introspective wisdom. It also involves acquiring and using interpersonal skills. This type of IQ grows throughout life
- Gaining freedom from senile dementias, including Alzheimer's Disease, and brain disorders such as aphasia, apraxia, alexia, etc., that contribute to mental health problems
- Gaining the ability to recall greater amounts of information from stored memory

Emotional Health

Emotional health relates to:

- Freedom from neuroses and psychoses
- Ability to have emotions and feel them, understanding that any emotion has both positive and negative connotations and consequences (Section #23). This ability to feel emotions involves neither conscious nor subconscious suppression or regression

Table 5.1

The 4 Levels of Health According to Western Systems Theory, Eastern and Western Psychology, and Religions

Spiritual
Emotional
Mental
Physical

Traditional Medicine Emphasis

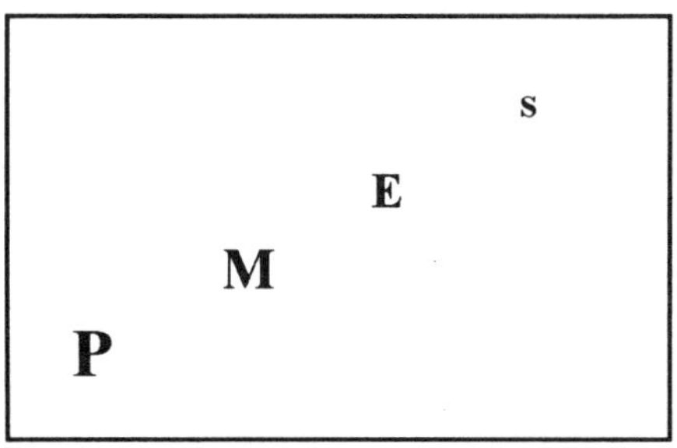

New Age Emphasis

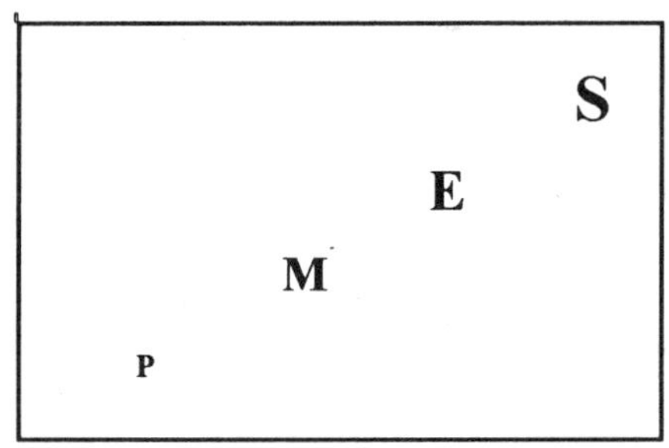

WHAT IS NEEDED:
Integration to Equal Emphasis

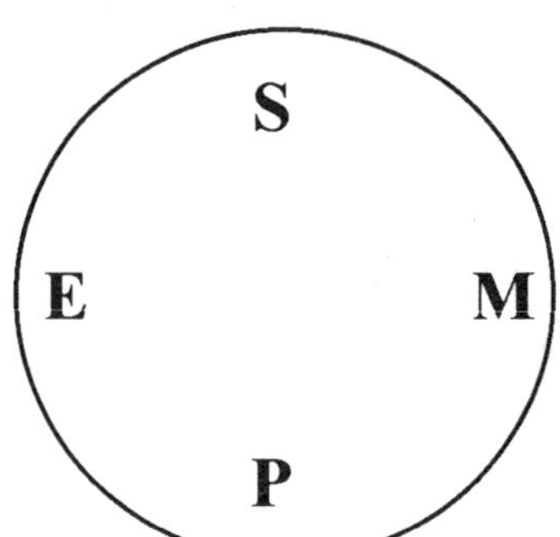

- Self-love, not selfish love. "I may dislike my behaviors, my actions, and wish to improve them, but at my core, my foundation, is my self" (Section #23 and Appendix D)

A major fundamental distinction must be made between mental health and emotional health. Having worked for eleven years in mental health administration, Swartz can state that the problems of the patients were primarily emotional in origin. We are so afraid of our emotions that we can't even classify correctly the subsystem of our healthcare system that is to deal with emotional problems. Mental and emotional levels interrelate (Section #23), but they are not the same.

Spiritual Health

For the authors, there is a distinct difference between the terms *religion* and *religious*. The former relates to formalized tenets, doctrines concerning the nature of man's collective ontological relationship to the universe. The latter relates to an individual's beliefs about a higher being and relationship to a specific God.

It is in this latter context that the authors place spiritual health. Spritual health relates to the person's individual belief system. It is not necessarily a product of any organized religion or belief system. Spritual health relates to how one perceives his health: i.e., "I am healthy" versus "I don't feel good." Section #23 deals extensively with this topic.

Systems Theory Principles

Rather than components of wholeness, the four levels of health may be considered strata of life experience and, as in systems theory, psychologies and religions, arranged on hierarchical levels. In systems theory, three general principles are in operation:

- More complex strata, or higher levels, cannot be solely explained in terms of lower levels. Lower levels are included in the higher, but the higher is greater than the lower
- Levels interrelate but are not the same
- The means of knowing and understanding the levels differ

Hierarchy. Matter can be described by mind, but matter cannot describe mind. Mind, in turn, cannot totally describe spirit. In the previously mentioned health example, the DNA of a cell in the breast can help replicate a female breast, given its memory encoding; the cells can communicate with other systems within the physical body, via neurotransmitters. However, the physical cell cannot know and understand the personality, the character, the entity known as Martha Thomas. Martha Thomas is aware of her physical body, its dimensions, weight, height, etc. She knows something is terribly wrong in her breast and is aware of at least some of the emotions connected with this knowing. Ms. Thomas *may* be consciously aware of her spiritual values; however, and all major world-wide religions would agree to this, she cannot totally know, comprehend, and understand God/All That Is/Supreme Being/Om. ("Collapse of the Hierarchy of Health", Section #7.)

Levels interrelate. One of the major contributions and advantages of psychoneuroimmunology (Section #14) is its awareness of this principle. However, the levels are not the same.

Skill levels. Because the levels or components are not the same, the means of knowing and understanding the levels of health differ. That is, different skills are needed at each level. Chemotherapy treatments are related to the physical level. One does not prescribe chemotherapy treatments as a primary means of reducing stress. Biofeedback training, hypnosis, relaxation training, and psychological counseling are all more appropriate means to deal with stress.

Practical Implications for Healthcare Treatment

From this explanation, it is clear that alternative healthcare therapists and traditional medical practitioners both want to cure or heal the patient. However, the means of healing differ. Too often, physical medicine and holistic medicine both mistakenly assume that the levels of health care are the same (Ref. #34).

Their assumptions are either that all is physical or all is spiritual. Means of treatment logically follow from whatever assumption they hold. If the patient is emotionally upset, give the patient a sedative. If the spirit permeates all, then spirit is nature. Therefore, we will naturally work with you via herbal medicines, massage, etc. Or, if your chakra (energy) centers are simply realigned, you *can* use your mind to cure cancer: just image it away naturally. Your physiological symptoms will disappear.

Considering the spiraling healthcare costs, including insurance premiums, and the lack of bedside manner as perceived by the patient, more and more people are turning to alternative holistic therapists. But many of these therapists, by ignoring the physical level, may be contributing to the spread of the disease. Consider this: one nationwide best selling book in the New Age market lists 313 physical problems, their emotional and/or spiritual causes, and what specific, cognitive affirmation will physically cure each problem (Ref. #53). For example, according to the author of this reference, AIDS is caused by failure to love yourself and sexual guilt. By repeating affirmations based on self-love, with self as a part of (not apart from) divinity, AIDS can be cured. Perhaps this author has not heard of having adulterated blood transfusions and contracting HIV in this fashion. Or, perhaps the author believes, as many New Agers do, that each of us creates whatever happens to us. So, if we deserve it, we will get it, one way or the other. Thus, if we have the ability to create cancer, we can uncreate it.

As many studies indicate (Refs. #13 and #114), all this creates is "New Age guilt". If they cannot cure AIDS, cancer, or whatever, this adds to feelings of hopelessness and worthlessness.

Both major camps collapse the hierarchy of human experience. In the domains of matter-mind-spirit, matter matters in terms of traditional medicine, the physical is all. In terms of many New Age practitioners, spirit matters, spirit is all. This leads to both camps competing against each other for the healthcare dollar. The patient in essence is told what to do by both camps: ignore or downplay the other. Both camps do a disservice to healing as a movement toward wholeness, wasting time and resources and escalating healthcare costs. If healing is a movement toward wholeness, physical disease occurs at one level, illness at another. Each level needs a different level of treatment.

Levels (or components) interrelate but they are not the same. Martha Thomas (this section's example) needs psychological counseling to come to grips with her physical diagnosis. She needs help in dealing with the emotions and stress associated with this diagnosis and perhaps even with the treatment (example: the stress associated with chemotherapy). She may need help, down the road, in coming to peace with herself if physical cure is impossible. The patient needs both the chemotherapy and the counseling.

Implications for the Co-Therapist

The patient as co-therapist, as co-manager - taking greater responsibility for his/her own treatment - needs to be aware, first of all, of the distinction between illness and disease. He/she needs to understand the impact of stress upon the body in terms of stress as cause of and/or contributor to disease (Section #17). Given this understanding, he/she needs to undertake life style behavioral changes, including stress management, that mitigate the impact of stress as well as the physiological progression of disease (Sections #18 and #23).

The co-therapist needs to understand the distinctions and interrelationships of these four levels of health, particularly being open to skills, knowledge, and resources that pertain to each of the four levels. The co-therapist should always be consciously aware of these questions and keep them in mind while undergoing treatment:

- To what level(s) are my symptoms related?
- Am I obtaining help and treatment appropriate to this/these level(s) of health?
- How might other levels be contributing to the problems I am currently experiencing and getting treatment for?

For practical examples related to these questions, the reader is urged to study Sections #6, #7, #17, #18, and #23.

If you, the reader, question the authors and the references listed at the end of this section on this point, consider this: Walk into any traditional hospital and ask to see the budget. What fiscal resources are allocated to physical care? To spiritual counseling? To psychological counseling? To patient education? Walk into a New Age alternative healthcare clinic. Ask at what point is the patient counseled to supplement natural healing treatment strategies with traditional medicine. The answers may not be surprising.

Finally, the co-therapist needs to understand some characteristics of each of these levels of health. Characteristics of spiritual health are given in Section #23. This level has been almost ignored in our healthcare system.

References: 13, 34, 42, 53, 58, 92, 95, 101, 110, 114

#6: TRADITIONAL MEDICINE: SUCCESSES AND PITFALLS

Successes

Western (or allopathic) medicine, for approximately the past 100 years, has emphasized *curative* medicine: disease interventions. The performance, on the surface, has been stellar. Among the successes of curative medicine have been:

- Technological advances, including:
  - Magnetic Resonance Imaging (MRI)
  - Positron Emission Tomography (PET)
  - Computer Assisted Tomography (CAT scanners)
  - Electrocardiogram (EKG)
  - Electroencephalogram (EEG)
- Immunization programs such as polio vaccination, pneumonia, chicken pox
- Bone marrow transplants
- Organ transplants
- Artificial hearts
- Research and development on the causes of physical disease
- Life-saving drugs
- Antibiotics
- Microsurgery
- Development of credentialing programs, standardized training, licensure and regulation of medical schools and professionals following the Flexnor Report of 1910, as supported by the Carnegie Foundation (Ref. #60)

  After this report, entitled "Medical Education in the United States and Canada," roughly 50 percent of North American medical schools were closed. Approximately 600 million dollars was spent to make medical education research-based and scientifically oriented. Henceforth, acceptable medicine (traditional medicine) was that which conformed to the rigors of scientific investigation (Ref. #60).

Traditional medicine can be distinguished from alternative medicine and therapies (Section #7) in this regard: traditional medicine is that which is universally accepted procedure in Western medical schools and teaching hospitals. Alternative medicine and therapies encompass those modalities which have not yet gained such acceptance.

Pitfalls

The emphasis upon physical health has been both Western traditional medicine's triumph and Achilles heel. The emphasis upon curative treatment of diseases has created problems in these major areas:

- Emphasis on physical health to the detriment of attention on the three other levels of health (Section #5)
- Problems with medical education
- Problems inherent in doctor-patient communication (Section #8)
- Allocation of resources - including technical and personnel
- Lack of emphasis on and reimbursement for preventive medicine
- Cost containment/prospective reimbursement programs
- Failure to recognize the limitations of allopathic medicine

Emphasis upon physical health. Physical health is only one level of health. A flourishing health system recognizes four levels of health: physical, mental, emotional and spiritual (Section #5) and the concomitant wellness programming (Section #18) associated with these levels.

One of the reasons so many are using alternative medicine therapists (Section #7) is alternative medicine's emphasis upon holism. It is not surprising that 72 percent of traditional medicine patients who are seeing alternative therapists will not tell their doctors they are doing so (Ref. #38).

Even within traditional medicine, disease is *multifactorial*. Disease can beget disease. Disease and its treatment can create other physical problems. For example, cancer treated by chemotherapy can cause nausea and hair loss. Physical problems in one area of the body can create problems elsewhere. Long term complications of diabetes include nerve and eye damage and cardiovascular disease.

As we age, the probabilities of each of us contracting multifactorial diseases increase. However, our society's emphasis upon physical health has contributed to a magic bullet single solution approach to disease. The answer is physical health. Within physical health, disease is caused by *a* problem. The latest magic bullet seems to be gene research. Within the next three years, this country will be investing billions of dollars per year on gene research; one estimate is $100 billion

(Ref. #66).

Finally, disease is also multifactorial in that illness accompanies disease. Illness is the stress and anxiety associated with disease. Illness is the patient's direct experience with disease. Too often, this is ignored by current traditional medical practice.

Problems with medical education. Medical education teaches diagnosis and treatment skills associated with physical health. However, problems with medical education (including those listed by doctors themselves [Ref #60]), include:

- The emphasis on basic science is out of proportion to clinical practice relevance
- Interpersonal skills with patients decline as medical education progresses
- Medical students get insufficient opportunity to interact with patients and few practice interviewing skills
- Patients seen are already in the hospital, their symptoms and diagnosis are already in progress
- Practice of early diagnosis, preventive medicine, or counseling regarding life style changes, etc., is uncommon. The person is not seen; the "kidney stone in room 201" is seen. In medical school, a student may begin seeing live patients in his/her third year
- Stress (Sections #17 and #18). What is ignored shall manifest. (See "ignorance," Table 23.1, Section #23.) Interns and residents, experiencing rigorous overwork and demand, themselves suffer from stress and anxiety, contributing to:
    - *Iatrogenic* (physician-related) disease and mistakes
    - Missed diagnosis
    - Errors in prescribing drugs and their dosage

  Such demands inevitably lead to callous attitudes. The patient becomes the "to do" diagnosis. Communication is curt.

Other problems with current medical training include:

- In training the highest priority is given to proficiency in technical skills, the lowest priority belongs to the humanities
- Intuition, a large part of diagnosis (as identified by doctors), belongs in the ethers of space, according to medical school culture. Doctors later seek ways to develop such ability
- Doctors would like to see the medical curriculum cover such subjects as nutrition, psychoneuroimmunology, alternative medicine, etc

Problems in doctor-patient communication. (The reader is also referred to Sections #8 and #22.) An aura of perfectionism surrounds the practice of medicine and the people in that field. The public, the layperson, hospital employees, and hospital administrators tend to "kowtow" to the physician. Traditionally, the patient views the physician as godlike and perfect, unable to make mistakes. The patient might leave the office suspecting that the physician made a mistake, but the public has placed physicians upon godlike pedestals. As Dr. Dossey states (Ref. #34), the myth of the all-powerful physician, benevolently using his/her powers to motivate the patient to follow the prescribed treatment regimen, contributes to the myth that we can become invincible to disease. We lose sight of the fact that physicians are also human beings.

Allocation of resources. Two major problem components are involved:

- Personnel
- Technology

Regarding personnel allocation, Dr. Leaf (Ref. #67) uses words similar to *absurdity*. He states that as long as the specialists (surgeons, neurosurgeons, cardiologists, etc.) are reimbursed by government and other third party payers at seven times the rate of general practitioners, internists, etc., then the ranks of the specialists will continue to swell, to the detriment of the generalists. Reports indicate that this country needs more generalists, i.e., primary care physicians.

Regarding technology, a 1993 editorial in the Pittsburgh Post-Gazette (Ref. #12) says it all: Allegheny County (western Pennsylvania, encompassing the city of Pittsburgh and its environs) has, as of the summer of 1993, only two fewer pieces of MRI (magnetic resonance imaging) equipment than all of Canada.

Lack of emphasis upon preventive medicine. Traditional medicine is perceived by many people as having failed. They are asking: What have we obtained with 14 percent of the Gross Domestic Product spent on healthcare? Our lives are longer, but at what cost and what quality? And is it true that traditional medicine has really improved our length of life, or is this improvement mostly due to turn-of-the-century preventive and public health medicine that produced a lengthened life expectancy?

For example, deaths and disease from common infections were declining prior to the introduction of antibiotics, due to public health measures such as (Ref. #81):

- Advances in agriculture in the 18th and 19th centuries allowed people to eat more varied and nutritious foods, increasing their immunity

- Water was purified
- Sewage disposal improved
- Milk was pasteurized

Thus the waste disposal engineer, the water works engineer, the food processor, and the farmer were as responsible as the doctor in eliminating approximately one fifth of the deaths due to infectious diseases.

Consider the fact that "Miles T. Gogh," born in 1842, surviving the infectious childhood diseases, could at age 45 (in 1887) still look forward to a potential life expectancy of 70 years. "Martha Marvel", born in 1942, could anticipate a life expectancy of 75 years. All the successes of 20th century medicine have not significantly lengthened the life expectancy.

The drug streptomycin, developed in 1947, was the first effective treatment of tuberculosis. It cut the death rate due to TB by 50 percent. However, approximately 95 percent of all cases had already been eliminated by 1945 (Ref. #81). Modern drug-resistant strains of TB have now developed and spread primarily due to a decrease in public health measures in our inner cities and overcrowding in our prisons.

From the above, it is evident that preventive medicine has done as much to prolong life as medical intervention. Should we be spending an estimated $100 billion on gene research (Ref. #66) to add an incremental extension of life expectancy while violence on the streets and in our homes drastically cuts our life expectancy?

Medical research, for example, has consistently demonstrated that coronary heart disease (CHD) is, with medications and/or life style changes, both preventable and reversible (Ref. #24 and #67). Yet there are very few referrals by physicians to this type of program that is well established and proven by research studies to be working. Furthermore, such rehabilitation programs are excluded from coverage by insurance programs. Dr. Leaf (Ref. #67) states that Blue Cross and Blue Shield will pay $30,000 for heart transplant surgery; but they will not reimburse a consumer for attending and completing a rehabilitation program costing a maximum of $2000. Medicare, according to Dr. Leaf, will not reimburse preventive medicine treatments at all.

Many times third party payers, the driving force behind how medicine is practiced, are "penny wise and pound foolish." Their pound foolishness contributes to the escalating costs of premiums. This in turn contributes to the high costs of doing business in this country and offers industry an excuse to relocate operations outside this country. It also contributes to the consumer diverting more and more of his/her net pay into healthcare insurance resulting in less net purchasing power. (Two-thirds of our economy is consumer-driven.) This situation leads to a lack of coverage on the part of the consumer. This lack of coverage was one of the major points cited in a national survey of doctors: 73 percent of U.S. physicians surveyed reported that patients' inability to pay for necessary treatment represented a serious problem for our current healthcare system (Ref. #11).

Perhaps this failure of third party payers to reimburse for preventive treatment is slowly changing. Mutual of Omaha is implementing a pilot program involving several hundred cardiac patients (Ref. #77). These patients would be reimbursed $3500 each for successfully completing the program designed by Dr. Dean Ornish to reverse the effects of arteriosclerosis (hardening of the arteries due to plaque build-up on artery walls). Program components include:

- A vegetarian, low-fat diet
- Exercise
- Meditation and yoga
- Support groups
- Assistance in stopping smoking

In contrast, bypass surgery generally costs $30,000 or more. Also, the effects of bypass surgery may not be lasting if the patient does not make the life style behavioral changes as represented by this program. (See "Preventive Medicine Research Institute", Section #31, for Ornish's program.)

Cost containment/prospective reimbursement programs. The Diagnostic Related Groups (DRGs) system (Sections #2 and #4), instituted in 1983, has put pressures on physicians to discharge the patient from the hospital after a short length of stay. Short, that is, compared to the years prior to 1983. The reader probably knows that his/her relatives and friends used to remain in the hospital up to two weeks to have an infant. Now, in 1996, it is common to stay in the hospital only 24 hours for the delivery process.

Physicians are stressed by the DRGs system. If the patient doesn't recuperate within the average length of stay, the physician experiences pressure from the hospital's administration. Why? According to the DRGs system, hospitals are paid *prospectively* for patient admissions, not paid *retrospectively*. In reality, this means that the patient has a certain number of days in which to recuperate from an illness based upon an average.

At one level, this system works. As the late U.S. Senator John Heinz, Chairman of the Special Committee on Aging in the U.S. Senate, stated in a letter to the Honorable Margaret M. Heckler, Secretary of the U.S. Department of Health and Human Services (Ref. #54), in 1985 the DRGs cost containment system has saved the taxpayer money while lifting the bankruptcy threat to the Medicare Trust Fund.

However, the major problem with this system persists to the present: patients may be discharged from the hospital prior to recuperation from their healthcare problems. A full recuperation may be difficult if the patient does not have sufficient skills, knowledge or resources to continue recuperation at home.

Limitations of traditional medicine. By focusing almost exclusively on the physical level of health, i.e., disease, almost to the exclusion of illness and its impact upon disease (See Section #5 for example), traditional medicine limits itself.

Another limitation relates to biomedicine's ever-increasing need to play catch with bacteria. Bacteria react to drugs by increasing their immunity to drugs through development of drug-resistant strains. This in turn necessitates more research to develop anti-bacterial drugs. An example of this ever escalating cycle is the resurgence of drug-resistant tuberculosis that has been manifesting in 12 states since 1989 (Ref. #28). Unless equal emphasis is placed upon preventive health, the only action remaining is to continually keep pace by providing state-of-the-art medical services, knowing that whatever treatments modern medicine develops, bacteria will counter it.

As Roter and Hall (Ref. #96) state, many medical symptoms do not fit neat diagnostic categories. Not only is disease multifactorial, with disease accompanied by its own illness (stress and anxiety), but stress and anxiety contribute to disease, creating the conditions for disease to gain a foothold in the body (Section #17). In different sections, this book cites studies demonstrating that stress and emotions are a major component of modern medicine. How can he/she counsel and treat effectively if a doctor is not trained in such matters?

Consequences. In systems theory, a system is as healthy as its subsystems. A healthy system is organic. It interacts not only with its subsystems, but also with other systems in its environment. A system that is organic is one that adapts to its environment. These are fundamental principles not only of systems theory but also of evolution and the science of ecology.

Healthcare reform cannot create a "healthy" healthcare system by ignoring the problems created by emphasis upon physical health or by ignoring the other levels of health that physical health interacts with: the mental, emotional and spiritual levels.

Healing, whether it be a person or the healthcare system, is accomplished when *all* components of health are taken into account.

References: 11, 12, 24, 28, 34, 38, 48, 60, 66, 67, 77, 81, 96

#7: ALTERNATIVE MEDICINE: SUCCESSES AND PITFALLS

Definition and Characteristics

Holistic medicine includes alternative medicine. It is whole (from the Greek, *holos*: whole) in that it accounts for the interaction of mind, body and spirit in both physical cure of disease and healing (Section #5).

From the connotations of the word *alternative*, placed in juxtaposition with traditional medicine (Section #6), it would seem fair to assume that alternative medicine would be out of the mainstream. However, alternative medicine practitioners would argue that traditional medicine is a quirk from the mainstream. Medical history confirms this. The ancient Greeks used treatments such as dreamwork - the interpretation of dreams as symbols of disease, herbology, light, nature, and sound. In the Middle Ages, the first medical societies (guilds) consisted of unemployed monks.

From 1500 through 1650, the Church slaughtered thousands of women who were thought to be witches. These were women who practiced shamanism, the application of the ancient healing arts. Henceforth, any woman was banned from the practice of medicine and denied membership in the medical societies. The New England witch trials in this country in the 1600s were a part of this movement (Ref. #1). These same healing arts have been found in all cultures including North, Central and South American Indian cultures and Asian cultures and religions. Thus from a historical perspective, traditional medicine is really a modern alternative from thousands of years of healing traditions.

True alternative *medicines* are complete medical systems. Chinese herbology, homeopathy, Indian Ayurvedic medicine, whether fully accepted or not, are specific and complete systems of dealing with health and disease. A fully trained practitioner of these systems might have as much training as an allopathic doctor. While these systems might treat any number of illnesses in strikingly different manners, in instances of emergency medical care their methods might be nearly identical with those of allopathic medicine.

Alternative *therapies,* on the other hand, usually deal with a particular type of illness or part of the body. They are usually not based on an all-inclusive concept of health and the body. An Alexander Technique teacher or massage therapist, for instance, would not purport to cure cancer (unless they were completely unscrupulous), but only to alleviate symptoms. Hence, most alternative therapies have more to do with symptom relief than physical cure, though some practitioners may claim otherwise.

Modern alternative therapies include body manipulation work, the application of natural remedies, mind-over-matter, life-style preventive medicine practices, energy exchange treatments. Appendix A presents a cursory listing of some of the more popular treatment modalities and a brief description of each. Some, as stated in Appendix A, have been more accepted by traditional medicine than others. (See Section #6 for a definition of traditional medicine.) Some are also used and/or based in religion, such as prayer, yoga, meditation, laying on of hands/faith healing, etc. Hence the practices or treatments span traditional worldwide major religions as well as Christian Protestant fundamentalist sects and the contemporary New Age movement.

New Age is an eclectic assortment of beliefs defying definition. Its ingredients include: quantum physics; mythology; a belief in reincarnation; assorted pseudosciences such as astrology; and a loose mix of Eastern, Native, Central and South American Indian religious beliefs and practices. Its purpose seems to be spiritual enlightenment of the individual living in harmony with nature. (This noble purpose is found in every major worldwide religion. See Appendix D.) The term, New Age, seems to be derived in part from the prediction of the Age of Aquarius, ushering in a new millenium. (If these words begin to recall for the reader a popular song from the late 60's, you can continue adding to this attempt at definition.) Within the realm of healing, New Age therapies can be found at the fringe of alternative medicine; these are least accepted by Western allopathic medicine. New Age healing therapies are included in the field of alternative medicine. However, all alternative medicines are not New Age. Many of these therapies are used to foster healing on all four levels but the spiritual level is the emphasis in New Age medicine.

The alternative medicine therapies, including New Age, listed in Appendix A have these characteristics in common:

- Physical cure
- The patient is a co-therapist

Successes of Alternative Therapy

Alternative therapy is big business. In 1990, the healthcare consumer paid an estimated $10.3 billion dollars for unconventional, alternative therapies. These were direct, out-of-pocket expenditures representing an estimated 425 million office visits to such therapists. This expenditure almost equals the total out-of-pocket expenditure for all hospital care in the United States: $12.8 billion (Ref. #38).

The reasons for these figures have to do with some of the pitfalls of traditional medicine (Section #6). Regardless of one's personal values, the reader has to respond to this financial figure as a success. Regardless of values, the reader has to regard the fact that chiropractic treatment ranks as the *third largest* primary healthcare profession in the Western hemisphere (Appendix A). People are using services provided by such practitioners. Furthermore, the National Institutes of Health now have a whole division devoted to clinical research on alternative therapies (Ref. #45). Even traditional doctors themselves use or refer clientele to these services (Ref. #60).

Why are people using these treatments? For the following major reasons:

- Empowerment
- The cult of health
- Pitfalls of traditional medicine

Empowerment. Patients report that they are tired of arriving on time for appointments and then having to wait for more than an hour to see a physician who spends little time communicating with them. They *want* to take greater responsibility for their own health, becoming a co-therapist. Alternative therapies and their practitioners offer clientele this responsibility, including the responsibilities associated with preventive medicine.

The cult of health. In our image-conscious age, appearances are reality. Fed by mass media advertising with emphasis upon the forever young, body beautiful, with the emphasis upon material consumption and "you can have it all," the consumer not only wants to be free from major disease but from nagging pain as well. A lot of the alternative therapies offer the consumer just this option without the costs associated with traditional medicine.

Pitfalls of traditional medicine. The pitfalls of traditional medicine have alienated people from traditional medicine and are driving patients to seek treatment elsewhere. For example, doctors are not trained in communication skills but in diagnosis. As costs continue to rise, people ask: "Can't my doctor at least listen to me?" Medical studies indicate that a general practitioner spends, on the average, a total of seven minutes with a patient (Ref. 48, Chapter 25). For more information on the pitfalls of traditional medicine, see Section #6.

Pitfalls of Alternative Therapy

For the authors, the problems and pitfalls of alternative therapy revolve about these basic issues:

- Research
- Credentials and training
- Blaming the victim syndrome
- Collapse of the hierarchy of health

Research. A great deal of research is done for those therapies and treatments more accepted by traditional medicine. (Appendix A.) For those modalities on the outer fringes, those furthest from acceptance by and incorporation into traditional medical practice, there is none. No research is done using a rigorous control group/experimental group/random sample design (true experimental research) having both external and internal validity and reliability.

What do exist are anecdotes. There are stories told by one friend to another. There are even pop media circuses, such as the myth that Norman Cousins was cured of cancer by watching humorous movies. This created the impression that cancer can be cured with humor. (Welcome to the 9.2 second sound byte age.) Reading Cousin's works gives an accurate description of what really happened and how humor contributed to the cure (Ref. #27).

For those modalities on the fringe and outer fringe, this lack of research is one of the reasons the traditionally conservative health insurance companies' benefits do not insure many of these therapies. Insurance company benefits are based on actuarial tables that compare disease rates of certain clustered demographic groups and treatment effectiveness to the frequency and costs of claims - to both their own and other insurance companies. Reasonable and Customary (R&C) tables are also used to compare physician charges for the treatment. Without research data, actuarial tables cannot exist. Without research, many physicians would not prescribe these fringe treatment modalities; without treatment description and use, R & C tables cannot be established.

One further note on research. As Section #14 states, the *placebo effect* can account for at least 30 percent of all physical cure. It is so prominent that clinical research must account for the placebo effect. That is, the results obtained must be consistent and must be due to the experimental treatment and not the placebo effect.

It stands to reason that if the placebo effect is so prominent a fixture in traditional medicine, it has to be prominent in alternative medicine as well. Martha Marvel does not acquire a new mind/body (Section #13) as she drives from Cardiologist Eva Hart's office and checks in at Herb Altee's natural New Age health spa. Practitioners of fringe and outer fringe, alternative medicine must also account for the placebo effect. They should be held accountable by the public, by the government, by the media and by market forces driven by the co-therapist. The consumer must ask: Where is your research?

Credentialing and training. It is interesting to compare the rigorousness of education, training, and continuing education needed by a practitioner in those fields more accepted by traditional medicine with those on the fringes. As a field gains greater acceptance, its practitioners need to expend a greater effort to aquire credentials.

Credentialing can vary within each field. For example, Swartz found one massage therapy association requiring 500 hours of training as a requirement for membership. Another massage therapy association requires only 15 hours of training. Therapists belonging to the latter association could potentially join the former; it was unclear to Swartz if one needed to acquire the net difference (485 hours) of training upon membership in the first association.

The New Age movement is a subculture. The same people attend the same conferences and workshops. Practitioners also attend and take each others' workshops. A specialist in Crystal Healing takes a workshop in Polarity Therapy or in Reflexology. (See Appendix A for descriptions.) In the name of holistic health, one must have knowledge in various disciplines if one is to be a holistic health practitioner. Unfortunately, the old adage is true: A little knowledge can be dangerous. In this case, dangerous to the health of their clients.

One more note: Where there's a quark, there's bound to be a quack. A quark is any of several elemental particles that are postulated to come in pairs of similar mass with one member having a charge of +2/3 and the other -1/3, and are held to make up hadrons (Merriam Webster's Collegiate Dictionary, Tenth Edition, 1993).

Any mass has quarks contained in it. Any mass or collection of therapies will attract quacks, which may be as difficult to identify as a quark. Therefore, New Age therapies are the quark of the more accepted alternative medicine therapies. Recall from above that alternative medicine is at least a $27 billion dollar industry. A quack can smell the dollar potential a mile away.

Blaming the victim syndrome. The down side of taking more responsibility for your health is this question: At what point does taking responsibility for my health become total control for all the events related to health that occur in my life? Taking more responsibility implies that I have greater control over my behaviors and my life style. At least I have choices and I have control over what I personally choose. Granted that mental processes and emotions impact physical health. Does this mean that I make myself sick? If I make myself sick, can I make myself well?

These are not esoteric, hypothetical questions. For example, Stephen Locke of Harvard has discovered that some cancer patients taught to use imagery (Section #26) on their tumors became *more* depressed from the tumors' reemergence than people treated with chemotherapy whose tumors recurred (Ref. #114). The patients were *blaming themselves* because they couldn't heal themselves. Hence, blaming the victim.

This raises many real questions. Telling the patients that they may not be successful in curing cancer raises the potential *nocebo effect* (negative placebo) (Section #14), destroying hope and creating hopelessness and helplessness. And yet, the thrust of much of mind/body medicine - and indeed, this book - is advocacy for the patient becoming the co-therapist. Many sections of this book were written to avoid this realistic mine/mind field. This pitfall is all too real if the focus of health is physical care. However, if the strategy is healing, on any given level of health (Section #5), this pitfall can be obviated. Both the healthcare professional and the layperson can benefit from Sections #5, #18 and #26.

The further away from traditional medicine, the louder this cry: "You create your own reality." This is the *cornerstone* of New Age religion and its health therapies. Responsible mind/body medical practitioners would say: "You *impact* your reality". Life does happen; i.e., we do not have complete control. (See also the answer to the question, "Why do bad things happen to good people?" in Section #23.) New Agers state: "Each of us creates our own reality. Each of us is unequivocably, 100 percent of the time, responsible for the events and experiences of our past, present, and future because of the thoughts we hold."

The feeling conveyed nonverbally by the New Age movement to the client on the part of the practitioner is this: "It is your fault if you are not physically cured. Your thoughts are holding you back. Remember, I am only the medium, the channel, the facilitator of the healing energy. You are the healer. You are the one responsible for your own health and your reality." It is as if they are saying: "Because you cannot physically heal, you are unenlightened." Again, the game of blaming the victim is played out, only this time totally irresponsibly.

What a no-lose proposition for the New Age therapist! This does away with the need for licensure, education, and training. Just your thoughts. Who can get a graduate degree and residency program in thought control? Why bother, even if one existed? Just your thoughts. This abnegates any responsibility for the New Age therapist in working with a client. This is not enlightenment.

New Age therapists of alternative medicine discredit the entire field of alternative therapy. They do a disservice to their clientele who innocently seek them out and look for answers. They do a disservice to the Joan Borysenkos, the Larry Dosseys, the Herbert Bensons, et al (see Bibliography) who have devoted their lives to alternative/holistic/ mind/body therapies and alternative medicine by discrediting their work. They do disservice to those practitioners in the fringe fields (Appendix A) who do advocate appropriate training and research.

Collapse of the hierarchy of health. Explanation of hierarchy and health as hierarchy is found in Section #5. Hierarchical collapse refers to the emphasis upon only one of the four levels of health covered in Section #5. Physical health is emphasized by traditional medicine almost to the exclusion of the other levels. As stated above this is one reason for people seeking alternative medical treatment.

Hierarchical theory is found in both Eastern and Western psychologies and religions. One of the primary tenets of all major religions is that the goal of humanity's evolution is growing back into Godhead (Section #23 and Appendix D). If God encompasses, permeates, and transcends reality, then God becomes ultimate reality. If Spirit is the highest reality to be known, then spiritual health is the pinnacle of health. Recall also that holistic health emphasizes the whole person, consisting of body, mind, and spirit.

In hierarchical systems theory, as found in science, certain laws are at play. One is that higher levels encompass those of a lower level (Section #5). Thus, spiritual health encompasses physical, mental and emotional health. With spirit being at the top of the heirarchy of existence, health becomes the ultimate goal of healing.

But at this point many alternative health therapists make one fatal turn away from known systems theory. In hierarchical systems theory, different levels interrelate, but they are not the same. Spiritual health interrelates with physical, mental and emotional health, but they are not the same.

Unfortunately, many holistic health practitioners collapse the hierarchy by equating spiritual health with physical health. They equate physical cure with healing, although the two are not the same (Section #5). Thus cancer can be cured through rebalance of energy flows, laying on of hands, faith healing, or whatever. Indeed, it is hard to distinguish New Age health therapies from New Age religion because, philosophically, for New Agers, the two are the same. Laypersons who hold these same beliefs will likely seek out New Age Health practitioners.

Such therapists also place emphasis upon therapies and skills that are more attuned to nature. This includes therapies such as herbology, aromatherapy, homeopathy, crystal healing, etc. Such therapists believe that if the skills are more natural, they are attuned more to God, because God is in nature. They forget that all major religions state that God transcends reality, being within and outside of reality (Appendix D). God is limitless. A limitless God is also found in the manufactured, synthetic drugs as well as in the natural herbs.

The very real danger here is that the holistic practitioner (by ignoring treatments based upon traditional medical research) is proselytizing in the name of holistic health - and possibly damaging not only the physical health but also the emotional and spiritual health of the client. If the alternative cure does not work, the client is left not only with the sense of worthlessness and emotional guilt felt in blaming the victim as previously discussed, but also with a deeper sense of spiritual guilt: "I am so worthless that even God has abandoned me. I must have done something terrible for God to punish me with this disease."

This guilt is created not only by New Age practitioners. Any religious sect that emphasizes the spiritual over the physical, mental, and emotional levels of health will create the same sense of guilt.

The very inherent danger of further damage to physical health also exists. For example, if we are saying affirmations, and using crystals and guided imagery to cure cancer, the cancer can be physically growing until it is too late to see an oncologist - even if the client could be persuaded to try traditional medicine.

Consumer Tips

Consumers do use alternative therapies. Again, consumer out-of-pocket expenditures in 1990 for such therapies almost equalled the total out-of-pocket expenditures for all hospital care in the United States (Ref. #38).

Considering the above pitfalls, the following are offered as critical points in seeking out alternative medicine practitioners (including practitioners of behavioral medicine interventions as advocated in this book in Section #18).

1. Ask these questions up front:
    - What are your credentials? Where were you trained? For how long?
    - Of what associations related to your specialty are you a member?
    - Will you refer me to traditional medicine specialists if you think it is warranted?
    - What is the research base for the claims you make?
    - What is the cost? How much is paid up front?
    - How long will it be before I begin to see the treatment work? What will I be looking for?
    - What, if any, side effects will there be? Herbs can be potent medicine, as potent as any synthetic drug
2. Find out if your insurance company covers any of the services. (For example, several insurance companies will pay a percentage of the treatment for chiropractic and osteopathy.)
3. Is this specialty licensed in your state? Why or why not?
4. Do you agree with the philosophy behind the treatment? As in traditional medicine, the client-doctor trust factor is critical for healing.
5. Are you willing to take greater responsibility for your own health? Are you willing to take the needed time to carry out prescribed exercises, diet, etc? If you cannot answer these questions in the affirmative, don't waste your money, your time, or the practitioner's time.
6. Beware of exaggerated claims on the part of the therapist, even though you may feel desperate enough to clutch at straws.
7. Beware of claims made by the therapist such as "God revealed to me the secret...." More often than not, this is the person's own ego masquerading as God, even if the person is sincere. And keep in mind: Where there is a quark, there's a quack.

References (Sources cited in this section): 1, 27, 38, 45, 48, 60, 114
References (Sources used as general reference works for this section): 7, 41, 89, 109

#8: HOW TO TALK WITH YOUR DOCTOR

Overview

Physicians traditionally have focused on a biological-based medical care. In this age of specialization, the psychiatrist is the one who specializes in the mind, the internist in the body, the OB-GYN in the female reproductive system. The health-care system has become systematized, fragmented and broken into bits. The parts have not necessarily been expected or encouraged to work as a whole. To date, only the specialty of family practice has been educated and trained to treat the whole person, to diagnose and intervene in healthcare situations. All people need a primary care physician. Levels of care are defined as (Ref. #48, Chapter 25):

- Primary (visits to family physician, general practitioner, and other general clinicians)
- Secondary (visits to a specialist and/or a stay in a community or general hospital)
- Tertiary (under care of a subspecialist and/or admission to an academic-oriented medical center)

Family practitioners refer to specialists, when necessary. Due to the expense of medical costs, many people will skirt the family doctor after they "diagnose" the problem and refer themselves directly to the specialist, assuming that the family doctor will refer them anyway. Unnecessary trips to the specialist increase healthcare cost expenditure. In order to maximize the effectiveness of his/her healthcare dollar: How does a layperson with a healthcare question, concern or problem begin to talk about it with the doctor?

A patient who perceives the physician as a time-pressured, overworked, curt, hassled professional always running behind, with an already crowded waiting room, may be intimidated to ask questions of his/her physician. In addition, the patient may have grown up with the admonishment to both trust and never question authority figures - particularly doctors. We must remember that the patient, as a consumer, is actually buying a service. Medicine is rapidly becoming more consumer-driven. The patient as consumer must decide on which product or service to buy and ask questions to help make appropriate decisions.

Communication Skills: Open-Ended Questions

Section #22 addresses the problems inherent in patient-doctor communication. It states that research studies indicate that only six percent of the time spent in communication between patient and doctor is used by patients to ask questions. Roter and Hall (Ref. #96) state that the majority of patient time is usually spent addressing close-ended questions posed by the doctor.

Section #22 also addresses the importance of open-ended questions for the doctor and how to ask them. Such questions elicit more self-disclosure and thus more information from the patient which the doctor can use in determining a diagnosis. Furthermore, they help the patient develop a rapport with the doctor. They are important in the patient's perception of satisfaction received, because the doctor is perceived as informative, dedicated and sincere (Ref. #96).

Open-ended questions asked by the patient have positive effects on the doctor as well. Roter and Hall (Ref. #96) report that doctors perceive patients who are actively engaged in conversation and ask questions, as being more:

- Intelligent
- Interested in their care
- Concerned for their health

Research on patients who ask such questions (see below) indicated that they perceive themselves as more in control. (For the importance of control, see "hardiness", Section #18.) This research also indicates that they did receive all the important information and did not fear being kept in the dark by their doctor.

Ask open-ended questions as much as possible. Questions that generally cannot be answered with either a yes or no answer are questions that begin with:

- Who
- What
- When
- How
- Where
- Why

What to Tell Your Doctor

Before you formulate your list of questions, answer this one: What should you tell your doctor? The answer is: nearly everything. You need to give your doctor all the details about your illness, including any other practitioners you have seen. Over 70 percent of the clients of biomedical practitioners who also see an alternative medicine practitioner for their major medical condition do not tell their doctor they are also seeing such a therapist (Ref. #38). The lack of communication could neutralize any treatment prescribed by your doctor and could potentially cause further damage. Telling your doctor "nearly everything " includes:

- Symptoms
- Drugs currently taking
- Past history of disease
- Psychological matters, including levels of stress and anxiety

Patient's Agenda: Questions to Ask

For the above reasons, as well as those listed in Section #4, the patient needs to become a co-manager, a co-therapist, in his/her healthcare. The categories of questions listed in Table 8.1 are pertinent to almost any diagnosis and prescribed treatment. Table 8.1 also summarizes the subsections below.

If you, the reader, feel uncomfortable in asking these questions when visiting your doctor, perhaps bringing a friend and/or caregiver along with you for support will help you be more assertive. Furthermore, he/she can help you record the answers (tape recorder, paper and pencil, obtaining written information and instructions, etc.).

If the doctor is truly busy and cannot address all of the questions, find out from him/her how to obtain the answers. In Swartz' own experience with basal cell carcinoma and sinusitis, many times the doctor's office staff and/or the pharmacist have provided the answers.

Visits to the doctor can be intimidating, embarrassing, fearful and/or anxiety-producing. You need to be able to communicate both your physical problems and your concerns to your doctor. Some of the questions you need to think about before you go are:

- What is it that *you* want to know when you go visit your doctor?
- What is your agenda?
- What do you need to know to take better care of yourself?
- What are the short term outcomes of your illness?
- What are the long term effects on your life?

Physicians, as highly educated professionals, are sometimes intimidating. If they appear rushed, the patient may feel rushed and forget the questions to ask during the visit. The best way to ensure that you receive all the information necessary to understand your situation is to take a list of questions when you see a physician. What should be on the list which will give the patient information needed to perform self-care skills? (See Table 8.1. for possible topics to discuss.)

Questions regarding treatment. Besides knowledge of medications, the patient needs to understand the specific treatment interventions the physician recommends. Whether a surgical or medical approach is indicated or suggested, the physician needs to explain it and the patient needs to understand it. Many times the patient makes decisions without having correctly understood information. The patient and the physician need to consider:

- Short and long term goals
- Side effects of the treatment intervention
- Risks involved
- Incidence of successful treatment
- Am I better off with it or without it?
- Is a second opinion advisable?

Questions regarding medications.
One of the major issues in patient education is patient compliance with prescribed medications. When a person can be taught, compliance is measurable. For example, many studies involving the proper techniques for the administration of metered dose inhalers demonstrate how few people actually learn the correct technique. Much medication is wasted, bronchodilation is not achieved, and the patient remains with shortness of breath.

If the patient receives a correct demonstration prior to a hospital discharge, greater therapeutic results from the medications would be observed. Cardiac medications and antihypertensives, vital to many people's lives, need to be taken regularly and the effect on the body carefully observed.

Reports in medical journals and on the national news media are increasingly documenting the problem of overmedicating the elderly.

In one example, Joe V. Alium was hospitalized after he drove to the local emergency room and said, "I think I am having a heart attack." He had, indeed, suffered a heart attack and he was provided with the customary medical regimen, including medications. Unfortunately he was over medicated and was "out of it for two months".

His son-in-law came to move him to the new state in which they now lived. Mr.

Alium had to be hoisted onto the plane, diapered due to incontinence, and was mentally confused. He was taken to a convalescent home near the family. The admitting physician discontinued the medication orders. By the second day of his admission, Mr. Alium was walking, unassisted, in the hall. Over the next few months, he regained his strength, energy and independence and he moved into the home with his daughter.

At an advanced age, he learned to drive again and passed his drivers test (written and practical). His last few years were spent enjoying his family and his newly found independence. Mr. Alium, in fact, never remembered what had happened those months of his life until he awoke at the convalescent home. Unfortunately, this situation is not unusual.

Although medications are often needed, they must be properly prescribed, administered and supervised. If healthcare providers expect patients to be "medication smart", then healthcare educators must teach patients and families what they need to know to be able to handle the responsibility. Medications have different effects on different people. Brand name drugs and generic drugs, although similar chemically, can be different and act differently. Generic drugs, although less expensive, are sometimes not the physicians' "drug of choice."

It is important for the healthcare provider to be aware of medication interactions. Some chemicals in medications adversely react with food or drink, causing increasing problems. All medications have some effect. No medication is considered truly safe. Even a simple pain reliever such as aspirin can cause stomach bleeding. In the 20th century, an inordinate number of medications have been developed for different illnesses. The pharmaceutical industry spends millions on research, development and production. The Federal Drug Administration investigates and approves medications before they are used for people.

Teaching and learning about medication becomes the responsibility of the patient and the healthcare provider. Local public libraries, bookstores, and medical libraries can assist the teacher and the learner in the search for knowledge concerning medication and treatment therapies.

Questions regarding finances. One of the areas that concerns patients is money, but most do not address the issue. Healthcare visits are costly. People are often reluctant to discuss finances with doctors. They may have the attitude that physicians and nurses, as humanitarian servants, do not deal with issues such as finances. Many times in the hospital settings, the healthcare employees do not know the true costs of hospitalizations. This may not be intentional. There are just too many tasks for the physician, nurse, respiratory therapist, physical therapist, nutritionist and social worker to perform for them to also deal with this issue. Traditionally, cost containment (Section #2) has been solely the responsibility of hospital administration.

Health insurance plans, managed care company plans, etc., determine policy and procedures and document such in writing. Patients need to read the information about their individual and/or family plan. Gone are the days when the consumer can blithely say, "My insurance will cover it." Regardless of the type of coverage and the insurance carrier, the consumer is generally held responsible for 20 percent of the balance of the allowable charges. It is imperative that patients become aware of such things as:

- Deductibles
- Premiums
- Coverages (in-patient and out-patient)
- Physician visits

Requisites Within Managed Care

In 1994, the Clinton Administration presented its healthcare reform plan to the U.S. Congress. The cornerstone of the plan was based upon "managed competition". Managed competition, mergers, and managed care, as cited in this work's "Pre-Publication Notes", are rapidly growing. Change, for better or worse, is occurring.

As costs escalate, the need for healthcare does not diminish, regardless of structural changes within the healthcare system. Furthermore, no matter what changes are recommended and instituted, patient-centered care needs to be adopted. We need to change our focus and urge the patient to take greater responsibility in managed care. The advice, guidance, recommendations and teaching given to patients by our healthcare professionals will help accomplish cost-effectiveness and the healing process in our healthcare system. Without the patient's input, our system does not function to maximum effectiveness.

Healthcare workers need to teach patients how to ask the right questions, to become assertive if necessary, and how to communicate fears, anxieties and concerns to make the most of their time spent with physicians.
Patients need to be considered normal, not aggressive or hostile, when they enter a physician's office with a problem. Time is valuable. Both doctors' and patients'

concerns to make the most of their time spent with physicians.
Patients need to be considered normal, not aggressive or hostile, when they enter a physician's office with a problem. Time is valuable. Both doctors' and patients' time must be wisely spent. Doctors should learn to listen and respect patients' time and concerns. All healthcare professionals and patients should review and enhance their own communication skills. This will mean money and time well-spent for both patient and healthcare provider.

References: 38, 48. 96

TABLE 8.1: WHAT TO ASK YOUR DOCTOR

(Note: The following categories are representative and are not meant to be all-inclusive.)

PREPARATION QUESTIONS:

- What is is that *you* want to know when you go visit your doctor?
- What do you tell the doctor?
- What is *your* agenda?
- What do you need to know to take better care of yourself?
- What are the short term outcomes of your illness?
- What are the long term effects on your life?
- Why am I sick?

DRUGS AND TREATMENTS:

- Why is this drug or treatment prescribed?
- What are the past rates of success and failure?
- Are their any side effects? What are they?
- What am I taking?
- When do I take it?·
- Are there any foods to take with this medication?
- Are there any foods to avoid with this medication?
- What signs of improvement should I look for?
- By when should I see improvement?

LIFE STYLE BEHAVIOR CHANGES:

- Smoking?
- Nutrition?
- Exercise?
- Other?

LOGISTICS:

- Office hours?
- Home visits?
- Secondary coverage?
- Therapists?
- Home healthcare?

FINANCES:

- Insurance coverage?
  - premiums
  - deductibles
  - coverages: inpatient/outpatient
- Payment schedule for uncovered portion of the bill?
- Physician visit charges?

SURGERY:

- Preparatory instructions?
- Procedures?
- Post operative complications?
- Success/failure rate?
- Credentials of surgeon?
- Experience of surgeon with this particular type of operation?
- Inpatient only?
- Outpatient options?
- Tests?
- Is the surgeon *scheduled* to do the operation the one who is going to *perform* the operation? Or is this person going to render technical assistance to others for "on-the-job" training? If the latter, do you consent to this?

SKILLS TRAINING:

- Make sure *you* know *how* to use medications prescribed, special equipment, etc.

DIAGNOSIS:

- Why this diagnosis?
- How did I get the disease?
- Additional tests needed?
- Second opinion(s)?

CLINICS/HOSPITALS:

- Ask for copy of Patient Bill of Rights
- Who is the Patient Rights representative?

Notes

PATIENT EDUCATION AND TRAINING

#9: COGNITIVE PROCESSING AND LEARNING STYLES

Overview

If doctor-patient communication is important within our managed care healthcare system (Section #8), then it becomes imperative to understand one another.

Cultural diversity within our nation is now a fact of life and helps create gaps in understanding. Diversity also exists within our brain, creating gaps in communication because of differences of perception. The brain has its own cognitive language(s) through which we filter our perceptions. The purpose of this section is to develop an awareness of these cognitive filters, how these perceptions are developed, how they generally affect the communication process, and how they can be better utilized in patient education.

Detailed information, references, resources, and examples (including those found in sections of this work) are provided for healthcare professionals and interested lay people in one assessment instrument measuring such cognitive processing and learning style differences. With such awareness, the communications process can be strengthened.

Cognitive Processing: Lateral Specialization

The human brain has two cerebral hemispheres and two portions containing the limbic system. Much of the human anatomy and physiology can be likened to a duplex house, in that a person has two (left and right) arms, legs, feet, eyes and hands. The limbic system is discussed in Section #16. The two hemispheres are left cerebral and right cerebral.

In terms of the cognitive processing, each brain hemisphere has developed specialized functions, called lateral specialization, perhaps over the last 3 to 4 million years.

Researchers have discovered that the specific cognitive functions of the left cerebral hemisphere include :

- Time orientation: processing information within a time frame
- Processing of events sequentially
- Verbal and written language skills

- Logic and rationalization
- Mathematics and sciences
- Analysis
- Convergent thinking skills
- Awareness of cause-and-effect relationships
- Emotions of happiness associated with perceived pleasant experiences
- Regulation of physical functions of the right side of the body (Figure 9.1 and Ref. #56)

Research has disclosed that the specific cognitive processing functions of the right cerebral hemisphere include:

- Processing of information in a timeless manner
- Processing of events simultaneously
- Visuo-spatial orientation
- Pattern awareness
- Imagery (Sections #11 and #26)
- Art, pictures
- Music (Section #21)
- Holistic perceptions and synthesis of information
- Divergent thinking skills
- The emotions associated with anger
- Regulation of physical functions of the left side of the body (Figure 9.1 and Ref. #56)

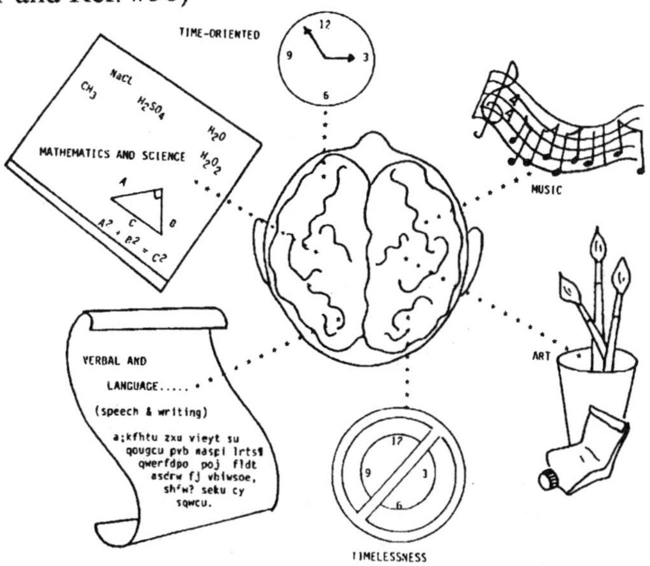

Figure 9.1. Left and Right Hemisphere Specialization

Integration of Left and Right Hemisphere Functions

The two cerebral hemispheres are complementary rather than competitive. Their coordinated activities are enhanced by the brain's physiology through:

- The corpus callosum, which allows the hemispheres to share learning and memory. It also unifies attention and awareness. Located between the two hemispheres, the corpus callosum is approximately 10 percent larger in females than males, allowing for increased rapid transit of neural (nerve) impulses between the hemispheres. Females can literally move ideas back and forth more quickly than males (Figure 9.2)

- The hippocampal commissure, which connects the two halves (rings) of the limbic system, enables the limbic system to coordinate activities (Section #16 and Figure 9.2)

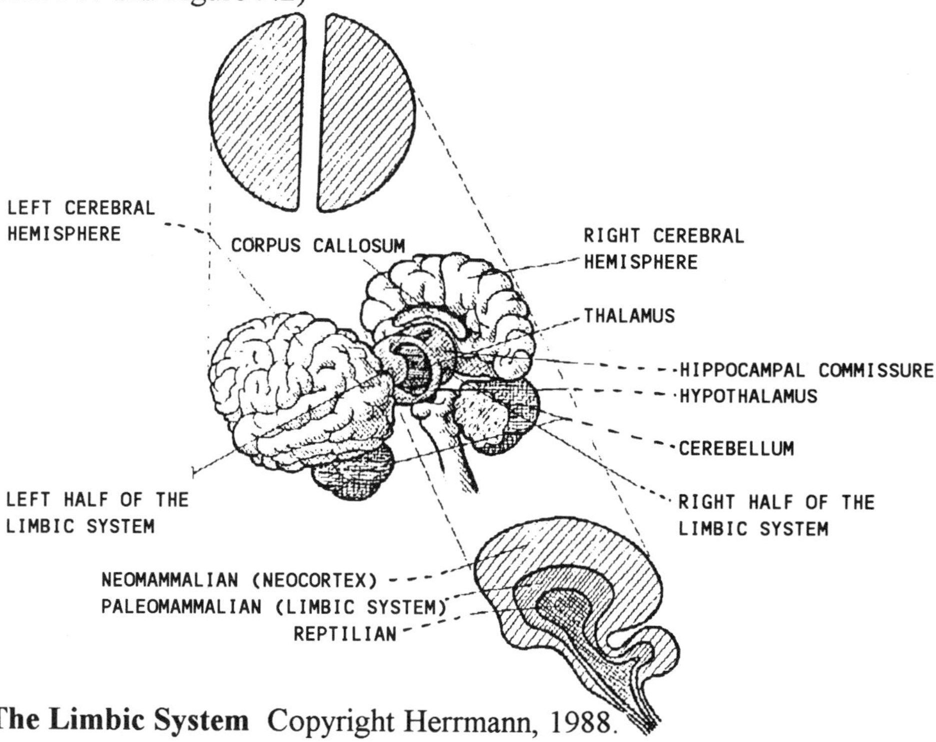

Figure 9.2. The Limbic System Copyright Herrmann, 1988.

Besides being intraconnected, the limbic system and the cerebral hemispheres are physiologically interconnected. Cognitive processing and regulation of somatic functions are interconnected with the functions of the limbic system: memory, emotions, and bodily functions (Section #16).

Dominance and Brain Dominance

Within this holistic web of interconnectedness, there exists the concept of dominance. For movement and position, during early childhood, human beings manifest a preference or tendency toward the use of one side of their bodies over the other. This preference is termed dominance. Examples of dominance include:

- Reaching out with one hand, arm, foot and/or leg
- Having one eye dominant over the other in terms of first focusing upon a visual field and then physically seeing the object(s) in that field

There are three basic reasons for dominance. These are :

- Society and culture
- Survival
- Physical effectiveness and efficiency (Ref. #56)

A child may have had natural preferences for using one or the other hand. Today, however, most people are right-handed. Why? Over the centuries of Western-Judeo civilization, natural left-handers were stigmatized. It was considered wrong to be left-handed. Only in the last few decades has this cultural taboo begun to be lifted. Consequently, left-handedness is on the increase.

Natural dominance preferences arise because of the brain's chief function: to aid the body in survival. Ned Herrmann, President of the Ned Herrmann Group (Section #31), believes that dominance enhances one's ability to respond both effectively and efficiently by eliminating a decision step (Ref. #56). For example, "What leg and arm shall I use first in order to get out of here?" The natural dominance preferences mean that one automatically reacts.

Herrmann also believes that dominance enables the person to hone his/her physical skills. Repetition and practice lead to effective and efficient gross and fine motor coordination and strength. This occurs well beyond what would happen if a physical appendage (arm, hand, leg, foot) were utilized only half as much.

Cognitive Dominance

A person has preferences in how he/she prefers to understand, to learn, to express (both verbally and nonverbally), to think, etc. These are termed cognitive preferences and this is what is meant by cognitive dominance. Cognitive preferences are the ones used for solving problems, learning, processing stimuli and information, etc. Examples are:

- Do we buy a car based on our "gut level feel" for the car or its styling, color, shape? These are right hemisphere preferences. Do we buy the car because of specifications such as weight; steering radius; estimated mpg, etc. These are left hemispheric preferences. (See the above discussion)
- What were my best school subjects? To what teachers and teaching methods did I respond the best? With what study methods did I learn and remember more?
- What profession(s) have I chosen for a career? (There is a direct relationship between occupational profile and cognitive preferences)

Individuals develop their preferred modes of thinking and learning styles from cognitive preferences. These can be measured. Persons who are aware of how they think and learn can adopt learning methods that fit naturally and match their natural learning style(s). Knowing this has tremendous ramifications not only for learning but also for daily communication, career development, and work productivity.

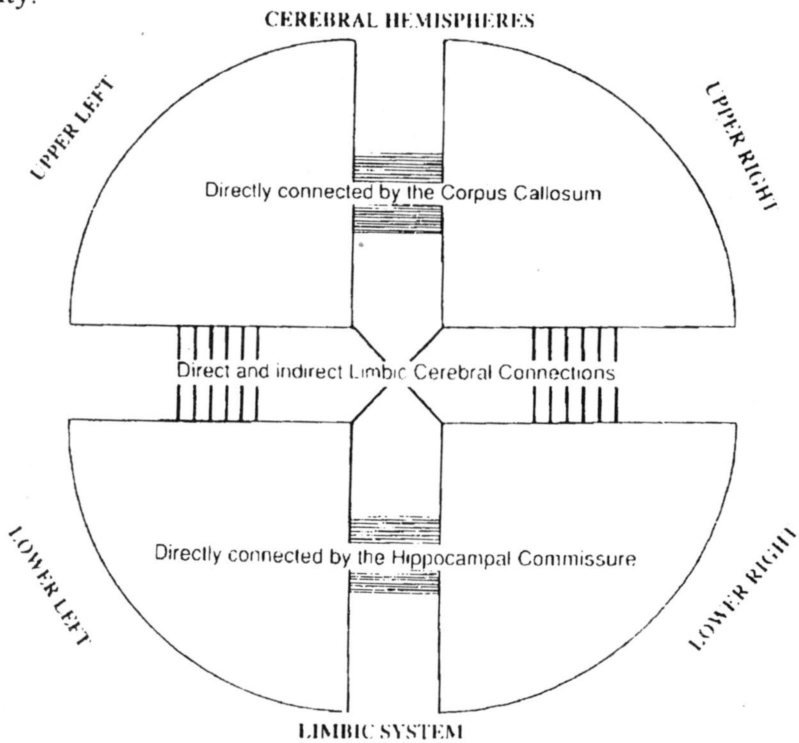

Figure 9.3. The Interconnected Brain System: Quadratic Model
Copyright Herrmann, 1988.

The Herrmann Brain Dominance Instrument

Several instruments have been devised to determine brain dominance and to assess cognitive processing and learning styles. The author recommends the Herrmann Brain Dominance Instrument (HBDI - Section #31, Resources: The Ned Herrmann Group) for the following reasons. The instrument:

- Has been researched thoroughly by independent professionals and organizations, including Princeton University's Educational Testing Service
- Has been assessed to be reliable and valid
- Closely approximates the Myers-Briggs Type Indicator, a popular psychological assessment tool
- Accounts for limbic system functions regarding emotions, information processing, learning and memory (Section #16)
- Has gained wide usage (more than 500,000 assessments through 1988)

TABLE 9.1 - BRAIN DOMINANCE: Definition of Terms

The following terms include, but are not limited to, those listed within the subsection, the Herrmann Brain Dominance Instrument, the four quadrants, as illustrated in Figure 9.4:

Analytic: Breaking up things or ideas into parts and examining them to see how they fit together.

Artistic: Taking enjoyment from or skillful in painting, drawing, music, or sculpture. Able to coordinate color, design, and texture for pleasant effects.

Conceptual: Able to conceive thoughts and ideas - to generalize abstract ideas from specific instances.

Controlled: Restrained, holding back, in charge of one's emotions.

Conservative: Tending toward maintaining traditional and proven views, conditions, and institutions.

Creative: Having unusual ideas and innovative thoughts. Able to put things together in new and imaginative ways.

Emotional: Having feelings that are easily stirred; displaying those feelings.

Holistic: Able to perceive and understand the "big picture" without dwelling on individual elements of an idea, concepts, or situation. Can see the forest as contrasted with the trees.

Interpersonal: Able easily to develop and maintain meaningful and pleasant relationships with many different kinds of people.

Logical: Able to reason deductively from what has gone before.

Mathematical: Perceiving and understanding numbers and being able to manipulate them to a desired end.

Organized: Able to arrange people, concepts, objects, elements, etc. into coherent relationships with each other.

Planning: Formulating methods or means to achieve a desired end in advance of taking actions to implement.

Quantitative: Oriented toward numerical relationships, inclined to know or seek exact measures.

Sequential: Dealing with things and ideas one after another or in order.

Simultaneous: Able to process more than one type of mental input at a time, e.g., visual, verbal, and musical. Able to attend to more than one activity at a time.

Spiritual: Having to do with spirit or soul as apart from the body or other material things.

Synthesizer: One who unites separate ideas, elements or concepts into something new.

Technical: Able to understand and apply engineering and scientific knowledge.

Source: A partial listing of definitions contained within the Herrmann Brain Dominance Instrument. Copyright: the Ned Herrmann Group, 1990.

The Four-Quadrant Model

Herrmann integrated the functions associated with the right and left cerebral hemispheres, and the right and left halves of the limbic system to create a quadratic model of thinking and learning. The foundation of this model, integrating the cerebral hemispheres and the limbic system, is illustrated in Figure 9.3.

Each quadrant of the whole brain/quadratic model of thinking and learning indicates a different information processing mode (see above) corresponding to the left and the right cerebral hemispheres and the two halves of the limbic system. This is represented in Figure 9.4. The four quadrants in Figure 9.4 represent Herrmann's developed instrument, the HBDI.

The four quadrants of the HBDI are described below, reading counter clockwise. Descriptions of the quadrants derive from the HBDI (Ref. #56 and Table 9.1: "Brain Dominance: Definition of Terms"). Illustrative definitions listed in each quadrant in Figure 9.4 are represented in the following descriptions of the four quadrants.

- Upper Left Cerebral (Quadrant A, Figure 9.4) The key descriptors for an Upper Left thinker are:
    - Logical
    - Analytical
    - Mathematical
    - Technical
    - Problem solving
    - Quantitative

  General profile statement: This person thinks in words and numbers.
  Overall profile descriptor: Facts.

- Lower Left Limbic (Quadrant B, Figure 9.4) The key descriptors for a Lower Left thinker are:
    - Controlled
    - Conservative
    - Planning
    - Organized
    - Administrative
    - Sequential
    - Procedural

  General profile statement: This person thinks in words and/or "rules."
  Overall profile descriptor: Form.

- Lower Right Limbic (Quadrant C, Figure 9.4)
  Key descriptors for a Lower Right thinker are:
    - Interpersonal
    - Emotional
    - Musical

- Spiritual

General profile statement: This person senses, "thinks" in feelings.
Overall profile descriptor: Feelings

- Upper Right Cerebral (Quadrant D, Figure 9.4)

  Key descriptors for an Upper Right thinker are:
  - Visual
  - Creative
  - Synthesizer
  - Artistic
  - Holistic
  - Conceptual
  - Risk-taker
  - Entrepreneur
  - Simultaneous

  General profile statement: This person thinks in images (Sections #11 and #26).
  Overall profile descriptor: Fantasy.

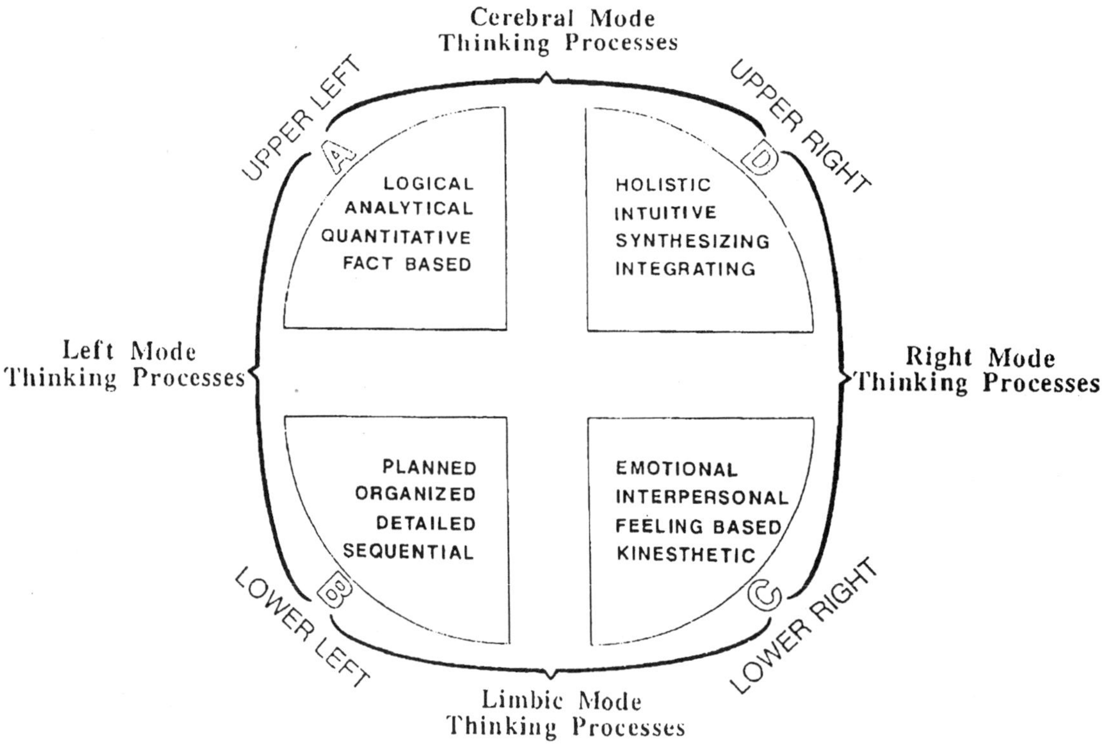

Figure 9.4. Whole Brain Quadratic Model. Copyright Herrmann, 1988

Assessment

For HBDI assessment purposes, the four quadrants are subdivided into three descriptive components, each of which is assigned a number range (1 to 3) on a continuum of 0 to 100 (Figure 9.5).

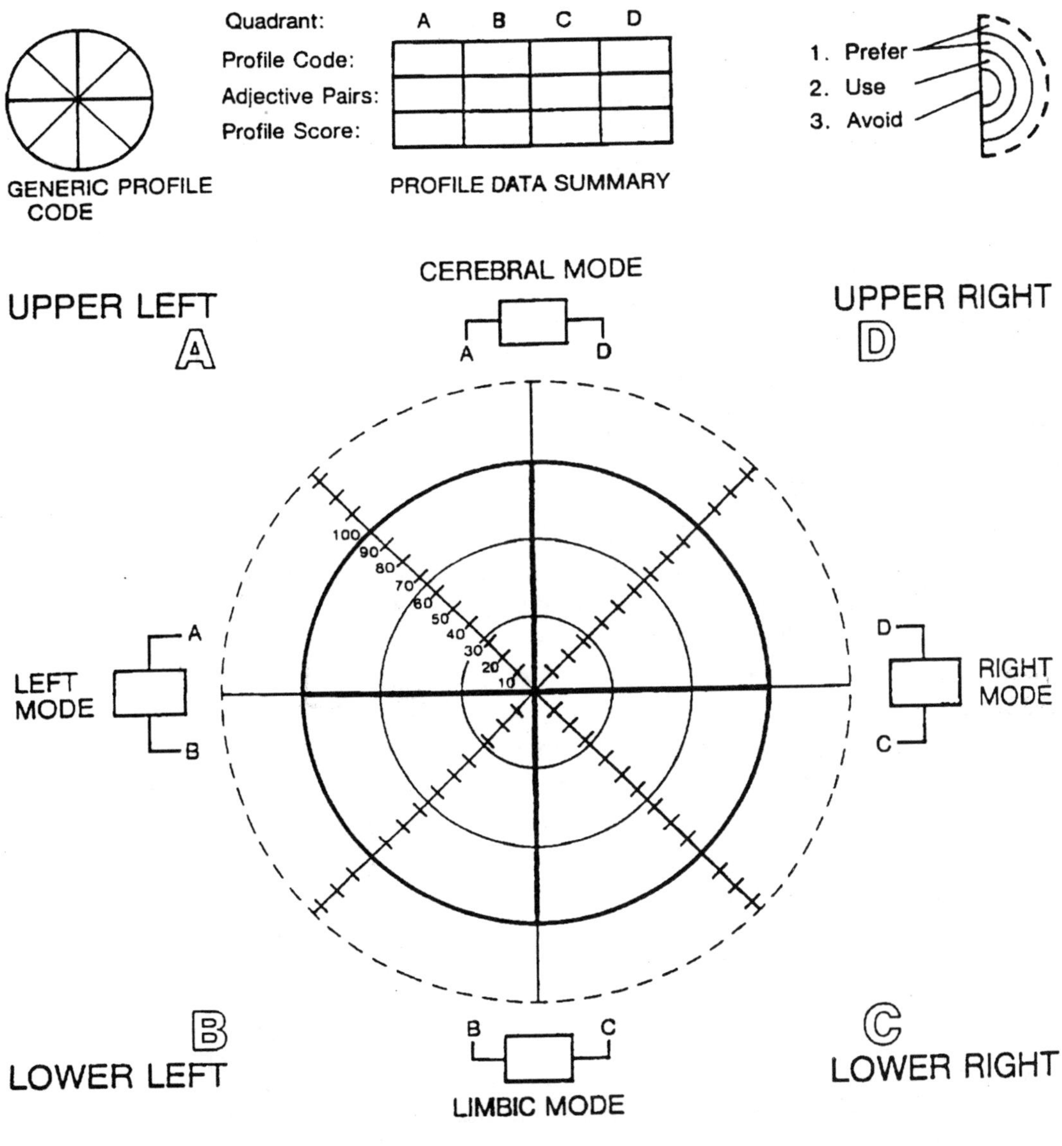

Figure 9.5. Herrmann Brain Dominance Profile. Copyright Herrmann, 1986.
Descriptions of the quadrant numerical assessments are:

No.	Descriptor	Statement/ Definition	Assessment/ Score Range
1	Dominant	I prefer using this mode of cognitive processing.	67-100
2	Use	I recognize the necessity for using this mode.	34-66
3	Avoidance	I will not use this mode of processing. I avoid it.	1-33

The HBDI should be administered by a trained, certified professional. The raw score of each quadrant, based on answers from the assessment instrument, is converted into a descriptor number (see above) for each quadrant; these numbers make up a four-number descriptor profile (see example below). Each numbered profile is read from upper left to upper right, counter clockwise. Subjects are then provided with narrative explanations of each descriptive number and an overall brain dominance profile assessment.

Figure 9.6 illustrates the HBDI profile of general practitioners,1-2-1-1. (See Section #30, Appendix B for a narrative description.) Recall that you read counter clockwise. Reading this profile from Upper Left to Upper Right, the numbers translate as follows: 1 = Upper Left; 2 = Lower Left; 1 = Lower Right; 1 = Upper Right. Because the probability that all general practitioners will have similar profiles is high, a composite occupational profile can be made by averaging the mean scores of all assessed general practitioners (one descriptor number per quadrant); a graphic picture of the score within each quadrant can then be drawn.

Representative listings of other health care professionals' profiles and their narrative descriptions are provided in Appendix B.

Additional Assessment Information

A few generalizations can be made regarding individual assessment:

- Value judgments are not reflected in final scores; each quadrant type has situational advantages
- Strong correlations exist between the individual's cognitive processing profiles and learning styles (Figure 9.7) with correspondingly strong

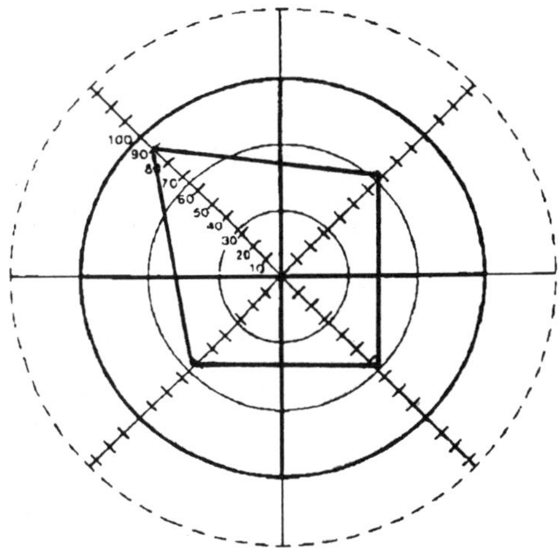

Figure 9.6. General Practitioner. Copyright Herrmann, 1988.

correlations between learning and occupational profiles

- In the U.S., quadrant dominance rates are approximately 30 percent for single dominance (preferring one quadrant only). For multidominance (preferring two or more quadrants) 40 percent prefer double dominance, 25 percent triple dominance, and 5 percent quadruple (no) dominance
- Approximately 70 percent of cognitive preferences are derived from environmental factors and 30 percent are innate, meaning that individuals can draw from nondominant quadrants to aid learning

Illustrative Application: Interrelationships

Communication is vital to the strengthening and maintenance of interpersonal relationships. The HBDI can enhance communication by identifying dominant modes of thinking so that individuals may better understand others' thinking processes and respond accordingly. (See Section 22 for examples of patient-staff communication.)

Illustrative Application: Occupational Relationships

In the same way that the HBDI can be used to enhance interpersonal relationships, it can be used to help coworkers understand each other and deal effectively with occupational situations. One example of increased understanding involves the

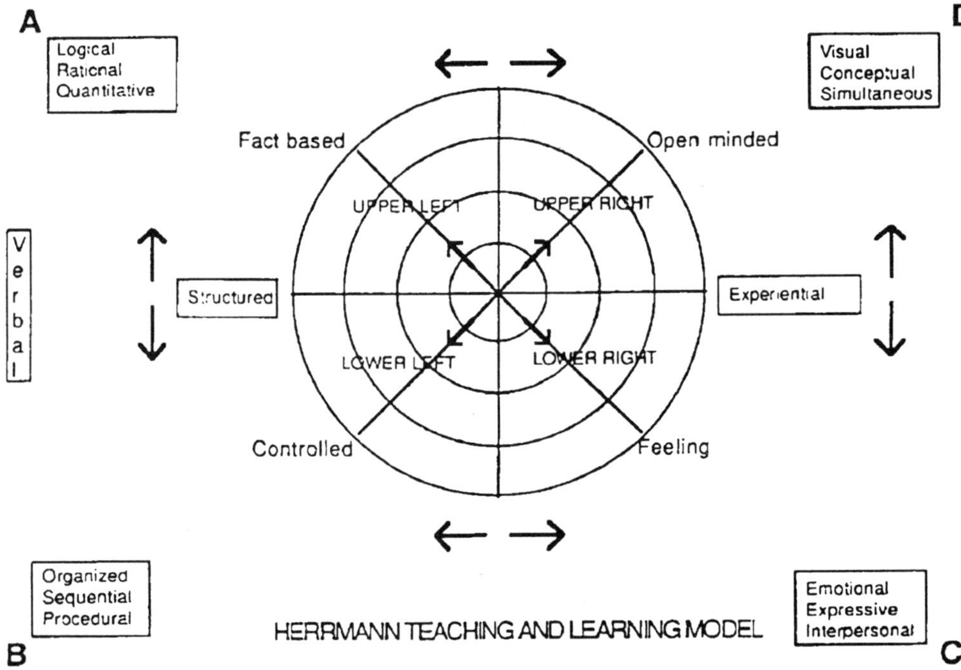

Figure 9.7. Whole Brain Teaching and Learning. Herrmann, 1988.

HBDI profile of school administrators in the U.S. Ninety-five percent of the school administrators assessed are lower left dominant, indicating their tendency to move very slowly, making sure that calculated risks are taken; and eliminating as much risk as possible before implementing school reforms - if they are considered at all. School personnel, parents, students, and communities may better understand why school system changes occur so slowly when they understand the mode of thinking of most school administrators.

A hospital administrator's profile is 1-1-2-2 (see Appendix B for a narrative description). What was said for school administrators above can also be said about hospital administrators. Refer to the example listed in Section #2, "other considerations".

Learning Styles and the HBDI

See Section #10. Also refer to Table 10.2 in Section #10.

Resources: For resources pertaining to the Herrmann Brain Dominance Instrument, see Section #31.

#10: TEACHING AND TRAINING

Purpose of Patient Teaching and Training

A common thread in education research literature is that the process of learning in life is continuous. Our past is the basis for the present; our present experiences are the basis for our future learning experiences. Individuals perform roles in life. Each role requires a knowledge base and skills as well as appropriate attitudes in order to effectively perform that role. A patient is a person experiencing a healthcare problem or crisis. This problem requires that the individual fulfill, appropriately, the role of a patient as co-manager or co-therapist, for reasons outlined in Section #4.

Patient education is an interactive process designed to meet common goals, involving both the client and the healthcare team. It is a critical component of continuity of care (Ref. #70) because it can produce positive life-style behavioral changes. Thus, patient education becomes a means of fostering healthcare promotion (Ref. #29) as well as wellness programming (Section #18), which includes preventive medicine. Patient education can meet these broad-based goals through teaching and training, which in turn address the patient's:

- Learning needs
- Motivational interests
- Abilities

Learning

As patients become partners in personal healthcare, the emphasis on patient education must include attention to the ways in which adults learn. Diversity in learning styles (see below), added to the lack of time the healthcare provider has to spend with the patient in the process of patient teaching, places stress on the family, patient, and healthcare provider. The current practice is that patients are discharged from the hospital with little knowledge of self-care. Gagne and Briggs (Ref. #44) have stated that learning involves change and growth in the individual; furthermore, the critical essence of learning involves change in performance. This implies behavioral-oriented objectives related to a person's skills, knowledge (intellectual and cognitive), and attitudes. Skills, knowledge, and attitudes are called *learning domains*. These learning domains involve the senses and concomitant psychomotor skills. (For a listing of the senses, see Section #26.) Hence, learning is a lifelong journey of growth.

Del Bueno (Ref. #31) states that an adult will be more motivated to learn if the content is presented with training methods related to the person's individual learning style(s). (For a detailed discussion of learning styles, refer to Section #9 and Table 10.2 of this section.) In his workshops on "training the trainer", Swartz places emphasis upon the learner, not the presenter/trainer. Salient questions are:

- What are the learner's beliefs, values, attitudes, and behavior?
- What is the learner's level of knowledge?
- What are the learner's goals?

Co-author Peske once had a patient named Mary. Mary had severe chronic obstructive lung disease and had attended a series of better breathing classes at her out patient pulmonary therapy center. At the demonstration of breathing retraining, Mary taught herself pursed lip breathing. A month later, having been referred to the facility for pulmonary rehabilitation, Mary told Peske she had been doing her pursed lip breathing. The significant social outcome for Mary had been, as she proudly stated, "That's the only way I can get up to my third floor walkup. John was going to have me move because my breathing had become so bad...pursed lip breathing has enabled me to stay in my home." A simple technique like pursed lip breathing provided the patient with enough comfort to retain the important things in her life. Mary was in control and needed to be able to make some decisions in her life.

As each of us learns in different ways, much of what we learn in situations is related to how we first perceive the information. Does the patient/client have the perception that the information is difficult? That, "I can't get it?" Internal dialogues may inhibit the desire to learn. Another inhibiting motivation is if the trainer (or patient educator) uses methodology or activities not associated with the subject content to be covered (Ref. #90).

Teaching methodologies that work for some patients might not work for others. Age in itself is not an impediment to learning but certainly decreased hearing ability and decreased visual perception, which often accompany old age, influence what and how individuals learn. Lack of time to teach and insecurity with the subject content influence the healthcare provider in the process of teaching. Other factors influencing the ability to learn include:

- Motivation
- Intellectual ability

- Past learning experiences

Narrow (Ref. #78) offers two additional factors necessary to consider in the process of patient teaching and learning. These are:

- Comfort
- Energy

When teaching adults, healthcare providers need to remember factors that have the ability to influence learning. The literature consistently states that age in itself is not a barrier to learning; what changes as individuals age is the speed or rate of learning. Adults learn best when:

- They feel the need to learn
- They have a sense of responsibility for what, why and how they learn

To summarize (Ref. #91 and #103):

- The learner is an individual with individualized needs, life experiences, and goals. Therefore, no two people will learn exactly the same information in the exact manner it is presented
- Patient education must involve the learner, creating an environment conducive to learning by paying attention to learning styles and methods appropriate to those styles
- Learning is growth and people can grow

Teachable Moments

The place, the time, and the environmental circumstances - these all affect learning. Learning can take place within any formal or informal setting involving individualized "one-on-one" instruction or formalized instruction in a group setting.

The first factor is the level of self-motivation on the part of the patient. The patient must be willing to learn. However, because of physical and psychological discomfort and stress, the patient may not be ready to learn until he/she is discharged. This is one reason why patient education studies have documented the lack of instruction by healthcare providers, including nurses (Ref. #31).

Hence *teachable moments* in learning involve not only individual variances in learning styles, the rate of learning, and intrinsic interest, but also the physical and psychological state. Patients may verbally express a need for knowledge and express a desire to learn but might be in too much discomfort to concentrate on what the healthcare provider is attempting to teach. The healthcare provider needs to be cognizant of such nonverbal cues.

Bedside teaching need not take much time. In fact, the most effective bedside teaching takes only a matter of minutes ***if*** the healthcare providers are aware that the attention span for learning new information (and/or skills) is short due to a lack of comfort and energy during illness.

In this environment, it is critical that the healthcare providers identify the most critically acute learning need and work with the patient to meet that objective. Such focusing upon the priorities is a second factor in effective bedside teaching. Healthcare providers also need to collaborate with one another to help the patient achieve needed objectives involving teaching, training and learning.

If patient education is to be effective rather than a haphazard "catch as catch can", it needs to be systematically implemented. Such a systems approach involves not only an analysis of what to teach and when to teach (Ref. #111), but also how to teach - the third important factor in effective bedside training. (See above; Section #9; and Table 10.2.)

The haphazard approach is due to many factors. (See "Barriers to Patient Education," Section #1.) Such factors include the lack of reimbursement to healthcare providers for patient education. (See "The patient education/cost containment research data base", Section #2.)

Healthcare providers are reimbursed for treating patients, not for teaching patients or for time spent with patients. If they were:

- We could have a more cost-effective healthcare system (Section #2)
- Patients would receive better care
- Emergency rooms would have far fewer visits
- Patients would have greater confidence in the system
- Patients would feel cared for (Sections #8 and #22)

It is time to begin to train the patient or the representative of the patient (the caregiver, for example) to be a co-manager.

Training

With limited resources in patient education, one of the greatest pitfalls to avoid is providing general information and documenting the effort as patient education. At this point, the patient, given his/her psychological state and associated stress and anxiety, may not be ready for or want general information.

This implies training - not broad-based education without a time frame. The difference between training and education is that training deals primarily with short-term, measurable objectives with behavior-oriented outcomes. Education involves long-term goals. A goal is defined as a long-term intent to accomplish a purpose. A well written training instructional objective has these criteria (Ref. #69):

(1) The end result or the crux of the objective. There is only one end result per objective
(2) Who is going to achieve the objective? Who has responsibility?
(3) The time frame - by when will the end result be achieved?
(4) The resources needed to achieve the objective
(5) Measurement criteria that clearly show how well the end result has been achieved

Training, more than education, addresses how adults learn. Adults are motivated to learn when the following principles of adult learning are followed (Ref. #63):

- The skills, knowledge, and values learned fit work or social roles needed in daily life
- There is a very short time frame from the end of training to the application of the learned skills and knowledge
- Adults need to work at their own pace
- Adults are capable of self-direction
- More learning is retained when it is reinforced

Such reinforcement helps insure that the learning is transferred from the training site (such as a hospital or rehabilitation facility) to the site where the learned skills and knowledges will be used.

Currently, behavioral outcome training is the most widely used planning system in education (Ref. #93). Training with emphasis upon behavioral changes obtains results. For example, review of research literature in patient education involving chronic disease indicates that behaviorally-oriented patient education programs are from 150 percent to 300 percent more effective than general educational programs (Ref. #93).

An example of a hospital-established learning center devoted to patient education and using the behavioral training model is listed in Table 10.1. For an example of training outcomes that this center has produced, refer to Section #24, "Patient Education as Social Support."

Cognitive Processing and Learning Styles.

Learning activities to meet the established behavioral objectives should be related to a person's cognitive processing and learning style(s). There is a strong correlation between a person's general cognitive processing profile (Section #9) and his/her preferred learning style(s). These relationships are depicted in Figure 9.7 and Table 10.2 of this section.

Such a match of learning activity/training methods and learning styles fosters communication and understanding. Table 10.2 matches teaching/training methods to learning styles.

Generally, Upper and Lower Left brain dominant learners need structure, safety and security to be incorporated into their learning processes, even experiential ones. Lower Right and Upper Right learners prefer experiential learning - learning by doing (Section #9).

Accelerated Learning as Training Methodology

The application of cognitive processing and learning styles is one method used within accelerated learning. Elsewhere, (Ref. #103) accelerated learning is defined as the art and science of the encoding and retrieval of information from the neuroanatomical brain. It is multifaceted learning involving all the senses (Section #26). A learning environment of being "relaxed, yet alert" is created.

Besides cognitive processing and learning styles, several of the methods involve mind/body behavioral medicine interventions, such as imagery, relaxation, and music (Sections #11, #19 and #21).

Within healthcare staff development, Pitt County Memorial Hospital/University Medical Center reduced its dropout rate of Registered Nurse applicants who could not pass the NCLEX-RN exam, the State Board licensure examination for registered nurses. The dropout rate was reduced from an average of 13.6 to 1.7, resulting in a net saving of approximately $192,000 per year [Ref. #80.]

In the South Jersey Hospital System, mean exam grades in the Basic Cardiac

Dysrhythmia segments of the South Jersey Education Consortium's Critical Care Courses for registered nurses when accelerated learning methods were used have been consistently higher than segments that were not taught using accelerated learning methods (Ref. #55).

In addition to staff development, there is a tremendous application of accelerated learning to patient education. Accelerated learning methods foster the relaxation response (Section #18), thereby reducing stress and increasing learning and long-term memory retention. Bu using accelerated learning, relaxation methods (the training methodology) are used to teach patients how to use and practice relaxation (the subject content). The "spin-off" effect is that accelerated learning fosters stress management programming (Section #18). These relaxation methods directly help the patient's stress and anxiety level - the illness accompanying the disease. Stress adversely affects learning and long-term memory retention (Ref. #103).

Patient educators can train patients to be co-therapists in the application of behavioral medicine interventions to their healing. In addition, patient educators can use accelerated learning methods, which incorporate mind/body behavioral medicine skills, to foster learning and long-term memory retention.

Table 10.3 presents a practical, sequential model using some accelerated learning methods. Accelerated learning is most beneficial when patient education is used as social support in a group setting - i.e., a group of patients are receiving the same training.

References: 29, 31, 44, 55, 63, 69, 70, 78, 80, 90, 91, 93, 103, 111

TABLE 10.1 PATIENT LEARNING CENTER

The University of Minnesota Hospital and Clinic's Patient Learning Center (PLC) provides a unique lab-like environment in which patients and their caregivers can receive information and practice skills needed for home care. The purpose of the PLC is to help facilitate a smooth transition from the hospital/clinic to home and to promote maximum independence and self-reliance for the patient and family. It was established to serve as a resource to physicians and nurses for teaching patients/caregivers the extensive, high-technology health related activities they will be performing after discharge from the hospital or clinic.

The PLC is open seven days a week and on holidays, and is staffed by registered nurses. There is a one time charge for the PLC that is covered by most patients' insurance companies. Patients/caregivers are taught on a one-on-one basis and may return as often as needed for additional review sessions. They may also bring as many caregivers as necessary to learn with them. Some of the units taught in the PLC include: IV medication administration, total parenteral nutrition, right atrial catheter care, IM or SQ injections, tube feedings, tracheostomy and laryngectomy care, diabetes skills, chemotherapy, and family life support.

Mannequins and simulation with the actual equipment to be used at home are used in the PLC. This allows patients/caregivers to learn in a more relaxed atmosphere with minimal distractions or interruptions, until an acceptable and safe level of expertise is achieved. Unit/clinic nurses provide follow-up by reinforcing the information taught in the PLC and by observing patients/caregivers technique as they practice the skills they have learned.

Source: Reprinted with permission from: Nancy L. Goldstein, MPA. See Resources, Section #31.

TABLE 10.2:
Learning Styles Represented by the Specialized Modes of the Four Quadrants
(The examples of training methods in each quadrant are not necessarily paired with the specific learning methods listed in each quadrant.)

LEFT

A-Upper Left

LEARNS BY: METHODS:	**EXAMPLES OF TRAINING**
Acquiring and quantifying facts	Case studies
Applying analysis and logic	Programmed learning
Thinking through ideas	Textbooks, biographies, resources
Building cases	Behavior modification
Forming theories	Formalized lecture

B-Lower Left

LEARNS BY: METHODS:	**EXAMPLES OF TRAINING**
Organizing and structuring content	Sequential order, structure
Sequencing content	Text books
Evaluating skills through practice	Behavioral modification
Implementing course content	Case studies
	Formalized lecture

TABLE 10.2: (continued)

RIGHT

D-Upper Right

LEARNS BY: METHODS:	**EXAMPLES OF TRAINING**
Taking initiative	Visual aids
Exploring hidden possibilities	Spontaneity/playfulness
Relying on intuition	Experiential learning: involvement
Self-discovery	Experimentation
Constructing concepts	Analogy/metaphor

C-Lower Right

LEARNS BY: METHODS:	**EXAMPLES OF TRAINING**
Listening and sharing ideas	Sensory movement
Integrating experiences with self	Role-playing
Moving and feeling	Music
Harmonizing with the content	Sub grouping
Emotional involvement	Interaction
	Experiential learning: involvement

Adapted from Ned Herrmann: The Creative Brain (Brain Books: Lake Lure, NC), 1988, p. 418.

Table 10.3 PATIENT EDUCATION: TEACHING/TRAINING MODEL

This model implements the principles of short and long term memory.
It is based upon R. G. Swartz'
*Accelerated Learning: **How** You Learn Determines **What** You Learn (Ref. #103).*

1. *Creating the Learning Environment*
    - Do basic relaxation exercises with the patients
    - Music
    - Imagery
    - Environmental stimuli

2. *"Active" Teaching Training*
    - Maintain the environment
    - Remember:
        - Your material encompasses an average of 20 minutes
        - The patient learns more at the beginning and end of the learning period
        - Your teaching needs to be reinforced by viable patient education materials in proper format. Focus upon the skills and knowledge that the patient needs
        - Present the material, verbally and nonverbally, in the patient's cognitive thinking/learning style(s). (See Section #9.) This is *important*
        - You may wish to use music during this 20-minute session (Refer to Section #21)

3. *Review*
    - The patient learns more at the beginning and end of the learning period
    - *Normally,* in the first 24 hours, we lose 80 percent of that which we've learned (Ref. #18). Hospital stays are not normal, adding to the stress (illness)

4. *Maintain the Learning/Healing Environment*
    Repeat basic relaxation exercises, combined with music & imagery.

Other Points:

1. Throughout these four steps, are you verbally and nonverbally contributing to a mental placebo effect (Section #14)?
2. You are not responsible for motivating a patient. You *are* responsible for creating a self-motivating environment. You *are* responsible for documenting the attempt and what was taught.
3. Again, properly formatted patient education materials will go a long way toward helping document your efforts as well as reinforcing the learning.

#11: IMAGERY AND LEARNING

Imagery and Learning

Section #16 presents the fact that one of the primary functions of the limbic system is its storage and retrieval of learning and memory, both short-term and long-term. Section #16 explains that the limbic system is where the senses are integrated.

A well known axiom in training and education is that the more senses employed in learning, the greater the learning. Section #12 and the information below deal with ways in which imagery is used to facilitate learning. Reference #103 provides other methods for using the senses in learning.

Relaxation is as important for learning (relaxed, yet alert, Ref. #103) as it is for healing. Relaxation helps the brain develop an alpha brain wave state which increases both learning capabilities (Refs. #84 and #103) and healing capabilities. Appropriate use of imagery (not just visualization - Section #26), combined with appropriate music (Section #21), fosters the relaxation response and the alpha brain wave state. (For a listing of all characteristics of alpha, refer to Section #19.)

Two important points to keep in mind are these:

- Imagery fosters relaxation which in turn fosters learning
- Imagery directly fosters learning and memory retention

Imagery Facilitates Recall

Ancient cultures used imagery (e.g., hieroglyphics) to depict their histories and beliefs. Currently, some educators advocate a return to these "basics" to aid recall, based on the research that explains the phenomenon.

An interesting aspect of imagery is that it occurs in the right hemisphere of the brain, an area that does not recognize time. (For a listing of brain hemisphere functions, see Section #9.) Though the events depicted through imagery may have occurred in the past, their associated images and descriptions and the recall of the events occur in the present. Thus, natural functions of the right hemisphere (imagery, creativity and timelessness: the use of past and present, as well as future) are doubly reinforced.

Application to Learning and Memory: Mnemonics (Memory Cues)

Although human beings think in images, they often are only paraconsciously aware of doing so. For example, when the name of a favorite football team is mentioned, a person mentally creates visual images and conjures up feelings associated with the team rather than creating images of the actual words used to describe the team.

Perhaps imagery was man's first method of thinking. (Early Grecians worshipped Mnemosyne, the goddess of memory, from whom the term *mnemonics* is derived.) Long before scientists knew of cerebral hemispheric specialization, the Greeks developed these major principles of memory retention:

- Imagination - using mental images to depict an association between new and old information
- Association - linking new information with old

Principles of Active Imagination

The more creative the imagination and the greater number of senses employed in imaging, the greater the memory recall. This tenet has been confirmed time and again and became the basis for the development of the principles of active imagination. These principles have proven to be effective in enhancing memory when applied in conjunction with the activation of the brain's natural functioning abilities and of the six senses. (See Section #26 for a listing.) The principles of active imagination are (Ref. #18 and #19):

- The more unrestricted the imagination, the greater the chance of memory retention. Images are more likely to elicit recall if they are:
    - Nonsensical
    - Ridiculous
    - Absurd
    - Sexual
    - Sensual
    - Bizarre
- The more colors used in images, the better the retention
- The larger the scale of the image, the greater the chances of recall
- The more specific and familiar the details of the image, the better the chance of associating new and old information and, thus, memory retention and recall. Abstract images offer fewer means of association. Specific terms should be used to describe images; they should be grounded in familiarity and consist mainly of words that easily form pictures in the mind

- The greater the incorporation of the six senses in the image, the greater the chances of recall because of the link of sensory integration with memory storage and retrieval via the limbic system (See Section #16) The powerful sense of smell, for example, can trigger many associations
- Learning involves self-responsibility. No person can tell another how to create an image or of what an image should consist. Every person must create images that are effective for him/her
- Order and sequence, structural requirements for left dominant individuals (Section #9), are necessary if associations are to occur. Images of new information must relate to the familiar (known information). The images of new information must symbolize specific items if the new terms or concepts they depict are to be remembered and if confusion is to be avoided. Keeping images simple also helps to avoid memory interference

Principles of Association

Principles of association that apply to traditional memory systems include:

- Using a key word as the associative link between new and old information
- Using order and sequencing techniques in imagery

Left/Right Note Study System

The principles of imagination and association can be incorporated into a study system that even more effectively enhances learning and memory retention. An important point is the format in which study notes are written. Note-taking should be formatted to coincide with the processes of each cerebral hemisphere and the bodily functions that each hemisphere controls. Because the right hemisphere is the artistic side of the brain and because it controls the left side of the body, images used in note-taking should be drawn on the left side of the page. Accordingly, because the left hemisphere is the language side and controls the right side of the body, narrative descriptions and key terms should be placed on the right side of the page. (This format was followed in examples given in Figure 11.1, examples 1-4.)

Why use these principles? Vision plays a major role in information processing. The right visual field of each eye is processed in the left hemisphere; the left visual field of each eye is processed in the right hemisphere (Ref. #56). This principle is illustrated in Figure 11.2.

In addition to using the Left/Right Note Study System for note-taking, it is an excellent tool for format of patient education materials (Section #12); for preparation of handout material; for staff development training; and for review of notes for test-taking preparation.

References: 18, 19, 56, 84, 103

Figure 11.1: Left/Right Note Study System

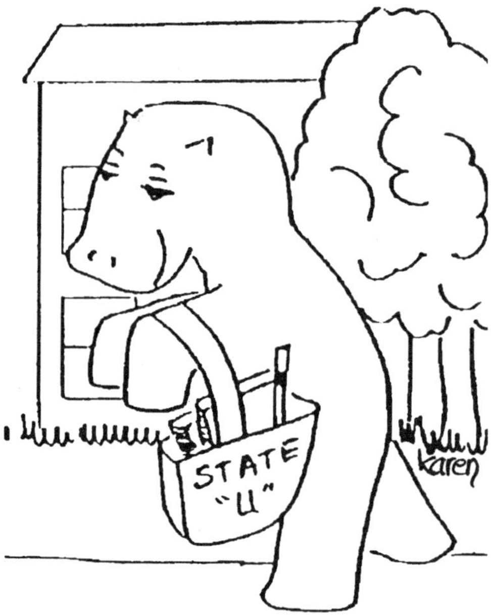

Example 1

HIPPOCAMPUS - A part of the limbic system used for learning and short-term memory.

(Be there with "Hippy." Talk to him. Ask him what courses he is taking. Feel his mouth as he opens his mouth to speak.)

Example 2

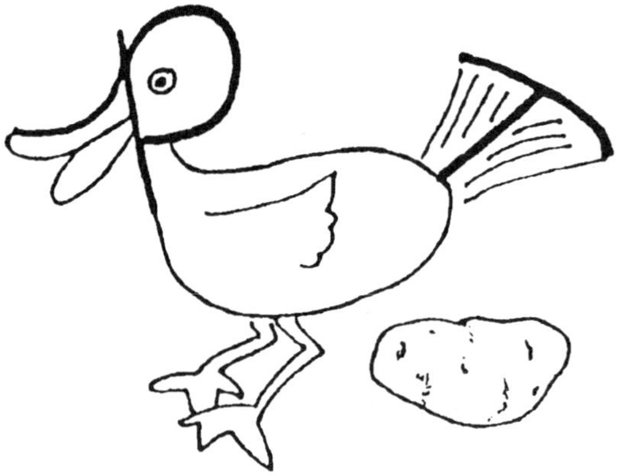

PATO - Spanish for duck. In language training, the Spanish noun for duck (pato) might easily be associated with a duck setting on a potato. The potato subliminally associates with "pato" and the image of the duck resembles the "p" and "t" of the Spanish term's spelling.

(Hear Daffy quacking as you step through the potato patch.)

Figure 11.1 (continued)

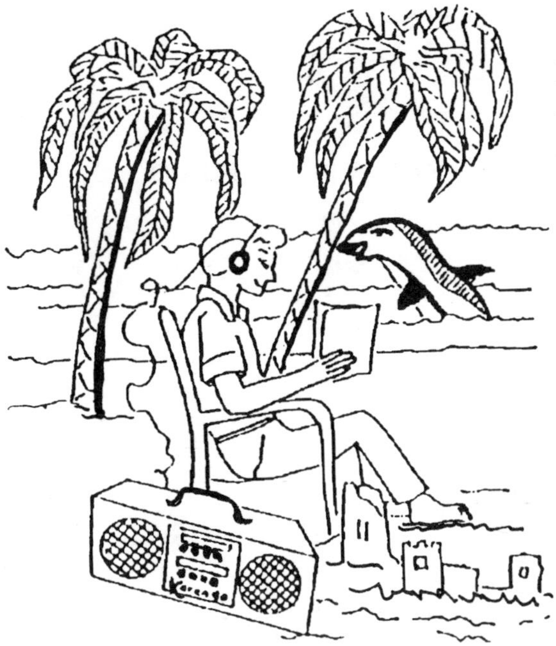

Example 3

LARGO - Classical music of a slow tempo ranging from 42 to 66 beats per minute. This music is conducive to producing the alpha brain wave state.

(Picture your favorite outdoors setting and hear the echo of the music as it reverberates through the scene.)

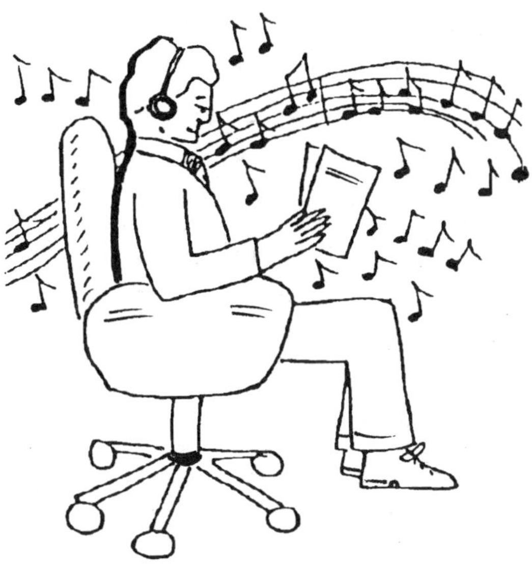

Example 4

ALPHA - The band of brain waves ranging from 8 to 13 cycles per second which is associated with "relaxed, yet alert" learning states.

(As you sink into the chair, feel the relaxation roll through your body and hear the calming music. As you read and comprehend the material in the book, put the book down and discuss it with Einstein.)

Figure 11.2: Book Format, Example for Left/Right Note Study System

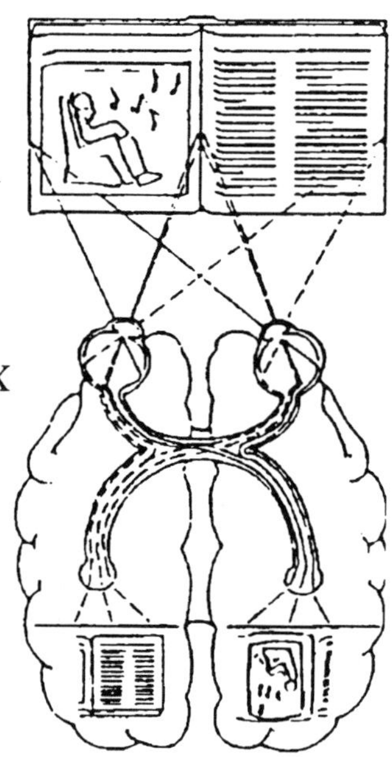

Modified from Herrmann, N: The Creative Brain. Lake Lure, NC: Brain Books, 1988. Reprinted with permission by the Ned Herrmann Group, Applied Creative Services, Ltd.

#12: DEVELOPMENT OF PATIENT EDUCATION MATERIALS

The importance of materials

Patient education materials are important for three reasons:

- Memory loss
- Training time factor
- Stimulation of patient interest

Memory loss. An adult learner normally loses 80 percent of the knowledge and skills originally acquired within the first 24 hours following such acquisition unless the learning is reinforced (Ref. #18). A person begins chronologically to take on characteristics of an adult learner in the ninth year of school (Ref. #63).

Three adult learning characteristics include:

- *Reinforcement and timing.* The acquired skills and knowledge (involving cognitive, affective, and psychomotor domains of learning) must be used as soon as possible
- *Meaning.* The skills and knowledge must be related to social or work roles needing to be performed
- *Self-direction.* An adult learner increasingly takes on greater responsibility for his/her learning (Ref. #63)

This memory loss is normal. The greater the stress, the greater the loss of learning, including even the ability to recall previously learned information.

Training time factor. The time available to train is low. Swartz estimates that a block of teachable moments involves 20 minutes average, given his informal polling of healthcare audiences in various places in the country. One study done by researchers indicated that doctors spend an average of 11 minutes with each patient while on rounds (Ref. #48, Chapter 25). Redman (Ref. #93) cites several studies attesting to the inadequacy of time spent on patient education, including the lack of physicians' time and an inadequate quantity of information given patients.

Appropriate patient evaluation materials (see below) address the time factor and reinforcement of learning under stressful conditions.

Stimulation of patient interest. Patient education literature from the last 15-20 years has suggested that written materials pertaining to patient education cannot substitute for patient teaching (Section #10). However, as Durback and Nendick (Ref. #36) have stated, pamphlets and other patient education materials certainly support bedside instruction.

Such materials fulfill the following functions (Ref. #36):

- They serve as a starting reference point for discussion between patient and nurse of the patient's healthcare concerns
- They serve as a take-home referral source for patients following discharge, reinforcing the learning process begun in the hospital

Tieney and Eisenberg (Ref. #105) state that materials can help motivate a patient to learn more about his/her condition as well as serve as a means of educating patient care givers about the patients' diagnosis and treatment process.

Guidelines for Development

The following guidelines are given to help the professional develop both teaching and training learning reinforcers as well as impart information in as "user-friendly" a manner as possible. (The professional is also urged to consult the Resources Section [Section #31] regarding how to obtain Section #5, "Producing Patient Education Materials", in the Patient Education Reference Handbook as developed by the Minnesota Chapter, American Society for Healthcare Education and Training.)

1. *The parameters of information.* Think like a patient. What is the information (skills and knowledge) the client needs to know and perform? A human services trainer has a National Brain Dominance profile of "2-2-1-1". See Section #9 for an interpretation of these numbers (see also Ref. #36). A trainer is cognitively "upper right" and "lower right" dominant (Section #9). An upper right cognitive processor has a natural tendency to think in universals, in interconnections, to see the big picture. For example, a client may need to learn how to use an inhaler. Understanding how stress contributes to asthma may be a secondary priority.

The parameters of information need not, however, be confined to strictly medical information. Refer to the four levels of health and the difference between disease and illness in Section #5.

2. *Language*. The information must be in user-friendly language and written on a fourth to seventh grade reading level. Under stress, both the professional engineer and the eighth grade dropout are equal in their ability to learn and recall pertinent information.

3. *Format.* The following format guide lines follow accelerated learning principles (Ref. #103) as well as brain/mind research into cognitive processing and learning (Ref. #56).

3.1. Textual elements should be placed as follows:

- Prose on the right side of a page or a book
- Art work (symbols, pictures, charts, graphs, etc.) on the left side of a page or a book
- Highlighted information (key terms, definitions, concepts, reinforcers, quotes, motivators, affirmations, etc.) on the extreme right side of a page or the right page of a book

This placement follows brain/mind functions, i.e.:

- The right hemisphere deals with visuospatial relationships, art, and imagery
- The left hemisphere deals with analytical and logical relationships

Whatever is seen with the left eye, physiologically connected to both the left and right hemispheres, crosses over to the right hemisphere. Thus, a natural function of the right hemisphere (imagery) is reinforced when information is presented in this format. See Figures 11.1 & 11.2, Section #11, for an illustration of this principle.

3.2. For the narrative presentation of subject content:

- Line lengths should be limited to six or seven words
- Type should be double spaced
- Information should be divided into smaller sections, if possible
- New or key terms, definitions, concepts, relationships, etc., should be highlighted, using different colors and type faces and/or separating them from the text for

SPECIAL ATTENTION

- New or key terms should be typed in LARGE PRINT; the larger the print, the greater the chance for memory retention and recall

- The type face for, and format of, words should follow the connotations and the mental images they inspire; for example, the word *relaxed* should be printed as relaxed, rather than RELAXED!!!
- Information should be repeated throughout the text to aid reinforcement

3.3 White space should be provided throughout the text to provide the reader/participant with space in which to create his/her own notes, symbols and images. Blank spaces should be positioned on the left side of the page.

3.4. Columns of information presented in charts, graphs, etc., should be separated from one another and/or from the text by space rather than by bars or lines. Bars clutter the text and place a barrier between related material, whereas open space sends a subliminal message that the material is interrelated.

3.5. New information should be presented in clusters of seven to nine items each, the number of items short-term memory most effectively retains.

3.6. Because retention is greater for items presented at the beginning and end of a block of text, the most important items in a cluster of information should be presented first and last.

References: 18, 36, 48, 56, 63, 93, 103, 105

THE BODY'S HEALING MECHANISMS

Notes

#13: THE INTELLIGENT BODY: MATTER MATTERS

Overview

The brain has been compared to a computer, capable of performing vast amounts of permutations as it stores and retrieves information. Computer programmers praise their efforts to create artificial intelligence and feel they are close to achieving parity with the human brain. At this time they are not even remotely close.

A computer can be programmed to handle any problem that can be broken down into information. But information is only one facet of a problem in the same way that physical health is only one level of health. (Refer to Section #5.) Perceptions and emotions are also facets of the problem. Values or ethics are another. A computer cannot be programmed to handle all the myriads of possible reactions a human can display (consciously and subconsciously) in his/her interactions. A computer works sequentially in time/space dimensions. With the brain and mind, a human can transcend time and space. An image of a future stressor, such as the rush hour traffic jam, can begin to tense up the body hours before, and after, the experience of traffic. A computer is a thing, an object that needs others adding to it via programming and circuitry if it is to evolve. The brain interacting with mind and body is an ever-evolving process capable of its own programming (Ref. #37). Within this process, a thing can become a thought; a thought can become a thing (see below).

The brain interacting with innate body intelligence in its millions of years of evolution performs three basic functions:
(1) Physical survival of the human body, the organism it is housed within, including the human body's health maintenance.
(2) Organization of the environment, with which the human being interacts so that the human being has a sense of coherence, meaning, and stability in life. This form provides the foundation of control.
(3) Growth of the human being in the physical, mental, emotional and spiritual domains.

This section is devoted to the dynamic intelligence of the body. The philosophical stream of consciousness is now empirical science. Understanding the dynamics of mind/body intelligence helps the reader focus upon his/her intrinsic healing systems. It is hoped that the reader will:

- Gain a greater appreciation for these systems
- Take greater responsibility in wellness programming so that these systems can be maintained
- Take greater responsibility in using both traditional medicine and mind/body behavioral medicine interventions (such as those listed in this book) that work in conjunction with these internal systems

Neurotransmitters

Neurotransmitters are chemicals created by neurons (nerve cells). They are released by one neuron through the microscopic gap between neurons, called synapses. They act as communication messengers among cells and between the brain and the body and become a part of the vocabulary of the body. (For a full description of such synaptic transmission, see Ref. #83.) The transmission speed of a nerve cell has been calculated at 225 miles per hour. For a message to travel from head to toe takes 1/50th of a second (Ref. #23).

From the 1920s through the mid 1980s, approximately 25 neurotransmitters were discovered (Ref. #87). Among them are:

- Adrenaline: involved in the body's metabolic functioning
- Dopamine: a chemical involved with a state of alertness
- Seratonin: a chemical involved with creating a state of calmness
- Substance P: involved in transmission of pain to the brain
- Norepinephrine: also involved in the state of alertness
- Acetycholine: a chemical involved with memory

The brain was previously described as a process. The brain has approximately 100 billion neurons - nerve cells. Each neuron has at least one thousand synaptic connections to neighboring neurons. Information is transmitted across these synaptic gaps. Such information is called a nerve impulse (Ref. #103). The fascinating thing about the process is that a neuron doesn't simply catch a signal from a neighboring neuron and pass it along in turn to its neighbors. It exercises choice. It can change the message en route, turning the chemical it received into a different one that it transmits (Ref. #23).

Neuropeptides

All the body's protein is produced from 22 basic amino acids, via the cell's DNA. (Ref. #71, regarding DNA, and below.) These proteins are linked into protein chains that can be further arranged into yet more complex substances called peptides.

Neuropeptides are chemical messengers made within a neuron (above); they are also found in other major organs of the body such as the heart, intestines, stomach, and kidneys.

Neuropeptides link (Ref. #20):

- The nervous system
- The endocrine system
- The immune system (Section #15)

Receptor sites (see below) for neuropeptides have been found on monocytes, a component of the immune system that engulfs invading organisms, communicates with B and T white blood cells to fight disease, and aids in healing of wounds.

Neuropeptides thus monitor a multidimensional information network. They both receive and transmit information as they themselves adapt to a changing environment. These are thinking, intelligent functions performed by the body, interacting with the brain and other major systems.

Positive Emission Tomography (PET) scans have revealed that a specific event, such as pain sensation or memory recalled, triggers a whole new pattern in the brain - at several sites simultaneously. Considering the neurotransmitters and neuropeptides circulating throughout the body, it has been found that the whole body displays changed patterns at the same time.

The body knows what is happening to it. Matter matters. The body is a web of fluid intelligence. Touch one strand and the whole web vibrates (Ref. #23).

Research studies have conclusively demonstrated that neuropeptides are associated with many mood states and states of physical being (Ref. #20). Among these are:

- Sexuality
- Appetite
- Pleasure
- Pain
- Learning
- Stress and anxiety

Since neuropeptides help regulate mood, they may help to integrate patterns of behavior.

The brain's limbic system (Section #16) has been found to contain vast amounts of these chemical messengers. This finding demonstrates a link between mental and emotional states and physiological processes.

Dr. Candace Pert, former Director of Brain Chemistry Division, National Institutes of Health, once stated that everything is interconnected at the level of the neuropeptide. She further stated that to arbitrarily separate mind and emotions from physical, bodily functions is bad science (Ref. #23).

DNA

Deoxyribonucleic acid (DNA) is the building block of life. All that makes you, the reader, physically human, all that you can do builds on the capacity programmed into one original molecule at the moment of your conception. As programmed intelligence, it is the basis of heredity and is found in every cell of the body.

However, DNA does not just work from programmed memory. DNA builds ribonucleic acid (RNA). RNA's mission seems to be to travel away from its DNA to produce the proteins that build and repair the body. Thus DNA can invent new chemicals at will, such as a new antibody after you catch a strain of flu you've never been exposed to before.

Science can account for only one percent of DNA activity. In this one percent, scientists have estimated that the number of molecular words (chemical vocabulary) produced in a single cell, if translated into English, would fill a 1000 volume library (Ref. #23).

The Inner Pharmacy

The incredible miracle of the intelligence of the human body is that the above chemicals and repair mechanisms are found not only in the human brain, with its capacity of thinking, reasoning, planning, problem solving, decision making, etc., but throughout the body. The body is a river of fluid, dynamic intelligence. One cannot distinguish a drop of water from the others in the river. One sees the whole, ever flowing. The body, at the chemical level, is the river - ever connected.

This fluid intelligence is the best pharmacy ever devised. Like the drug companies, it produces diuretics, tranquilizers, sleeping pills, antibodies, pain pills, etc. But the body produces better internal drugs (Ref. #81):

- Side effects are minimal or nonexistent

- The dosage is always correct
- The dosage is always given on time
- As part of this internal intelligence, the directions for taking it are contained in the drug itself

The Body Prescribes Patient Education to Itself

A key to the body's pharmacy is the receptor, a molecular structure found on every cell in the body. Any given cell may contain hundreds or even thousands of different types of receptors, found on the surface of the cell membrane. Each receptor type has a specific three-dimensional shape. It is the lock for the chemical key with the corresponding shape. Each neurotransmitter or neuropeptide has a specific shape (the key) that can only fit a corresponding receptor shape (the lock). When the receptor and chemical are fitted, once the key is in the lock, the activity of that cell is either inhibited or stimulated (Ref. #81).

The human body had millennia of research and development and trial and error to perfect this system. When disease breaks down the body's health maintenance systems and artificial drugs have to be used, drugs stimulate the body's natural processes because they simulate the shape of the body's natural substances. They also correspond to the keys for the locks.

Incidentally, pharmacological research and development should have their due. Modern drug companies do not have millennia, ethical considerations preclude evolution's weeding out process for the survival of the fittest. Hitting the correct cell receptor, minimizing the side effects, and maximizing the effectiveness and efficiency of the correct dosage is a different process, not unlike planning a manned space flight to the moon.

An Example: the Natural Pain Killer

Natural pain killer receptor sites in the brain were discovered by Johns Hopkins University and University of Aberdeen researchers in 1975. They isolated a substance that had the same properties as the artificial drug morphine, known as an effective pain killer for severe pain. Researchers called this substance enkophalin - meaning in the head. (The active ingredient of enkophalin is a mixture of two peptide molecules [Ref. #81]).

Enkophalins are the receptor sites alluded to above. The researchers further reasoned that if the receptor sites, the locks, exist then natural keys to these locks must also exist. These natural keys were/are the brain's natural pain killers - the endorphins that are endogenous morphines (Ref. #81).

Since 1975, opiates have been discovered in the endorphin family. One of these, dynophrin, is almost 200 times stronger than morphine as a pain killer (Ref. #81). Researchers have consistently discovered that the enkophalins and endorphins (Ref. #81):

- Relieve pain
- Reduce anxiety
- Induce pleasure
- Can be addictive
- Enhance immune system function (Section #15)
- Can be activated by the placebo effect (Section #14)

Regarding addiction, researchers have unfortunately also discovered that, like the synthetic opiate drugs such as opium and heroin, the natural opiates can also be addictive. It appears any substance that acts as the key to fit the lock (the receptor site) that spurs cell activity, reduces pain, and induces pleasure, can be addictive.

Why would the body develop such natural opiates? In a word, survival. If faced with an immediate threat to its existence, the body activates the "fight or flight response" (Section #18). A natural pain killer would reduce pain sensation to allow the body to better cope with the immediate threat to its survival.

This natural pain killer system is also activated by *placebos*. Placebos (Section #14) are inert substances with no cause-and-effect pharmacological properties. Research has shown that the placebo effect accounts for at least three percent of healing in all drug and surgical procedures (Refs. #48, #57, and #81). The belief on the part of the patient regarding the placebo is what triggers the patient's body to produce the needed chemicals, such as the endorphins, that cause the healing to take place.

References: 20, 23, 37, 48, 57, 71, 81, 83, 87, 103

Additional Reading: For a more complete description of the neuroanatomical brain and its communication, in lay person's language, see Ref. #83 and Ref. #103. For a description of the brain's ability to form chemical patterns and its implications for healthcare and patient education, consult Section #9 and Ref. #103.

#14: PSYCHONEUROIMMUNOLOGY

Definition

Psychoneuroimmunology (PNI) is a field of medical science investigating the interaction of the mind (psycho), body (the neuroendocrine system, consisting of the nervous system and the hormonal system), and the immune system (Section #15). Another emerging name for this is mind/body medicine.

In Section #13, the reader was introduced to mind/body medicine in terms of the innate, dynamic intelligence that the body itself possesses. Technically, PNI is really the interaction of human mind (including emotions and spirit) with the physical mind/body, producing mind-mind/body medicine. However, for purposes of simplification, references to mind-mind/body medicine will, in this book, use the more popular terms of either PNI or mind/body medicine to refer to both levels of mind: the mental human mind and the physical body's intelligence.

History: Two Landmark Studies

In 1974, at the University of Rochester's School of Medicine and Dentistry, psychologist Robert Adler performed what is now regarded as a landmark experiment. Adler conditioned the immune system of white rats to respond solely to water flavored with saccharin, as if they were responding to a drug, cyclophosphamide, which decreased the number of T-cells (Section #15) in their blood stream. This was classical Pavlovian conditioning: stimulus and response. The immune system could learn, could be conditioned, just as Pavlov's dogs were conditioned to salivate at the sound of a bell (Ref. #48, Chapter 1).

Up to this time, scientists believed that the brain and the immune system were separate entities, with no influence upon the other. Adler's and other subsequent experiments began to uncover more links between the brain, the central nervous system, and the immune system.

Another landmark study was begun in the late 1970's by Dr. David Spiegel, a psychiatrist at Stanford University (Ref. #48, Chapter 20). If there are physiological links, does that mean that the human mind can influence physiological disease?

Dr. Spiegel intended to prove that women with advanced, metastisized breast cancer (spread throughout the body) would suffer less from the illness (the emotional distress accompanying the disease - Section #5), if placed at random in social support groups, than those women not placed. This was proven. Quality of life of these women did improve. He wanted also to consciously disprove the hypothesis that mental and emotional factors influence the course of cancer. However, what he discovered was that the women in the support groups lived an average of 18 months longer. Collectively, this was not their medical prognosis, given the advanced stage of their disease.

Research Evidence for PNI

Medical research must by nature be conservative. After all, it deals with people's lives. The results must be as clear as possible in terms of these three criteria:

- Objectivity (unbiased)
- Ability to be replicated in subsequent experiments performed by different researchers
- Elimination of chance

Results are generally considered significant, if statistically they could occur by chance five or fewer times out of 100 studies.

The medical research for the existence of PNI comes from three basic categories :

- Clinical research
- Epidemiological research
- Physiological research (Ref. #48, Chapter 1)

Clinical research tests the effectiveness of mind/body medicine in preventing and/or alleviating the symptoms of, and/or treating, specific diseases. An example would be the Spiegel research cited above.

Epidemiological research tests the relationships between certain psychological factors and certain diseases in the population at large. An example would be the relationship of hostility to cardiovascular disease. (There is a positive relationship: hostility raises the body's stress hormone levels, which in turn can raise blood cholesterol levels, which in turn contribute to atherosclerosis [blockages in the arteries caused by a build up of plaque], thus creating coronary heart disease.)

Physiological research investigates the biological (neurotransmitter links among the brain and the body's chemical neuropeptide, etc.) and immune systems (Sections #13 and #15).

The Placebo Effect

Placebo (Latin): "I shall please."

The placebo effect can be defined as obtaining a physiological action or effect on a disorder for which the placebo prescribed contained no active ingredients designed to treat that disorder. The inert sugar pill is the typical example. Furthermore, the patients for whom they are prescribed typically do not know that they are receiving placebos.

Since the 1950s, medical research has indicated that the placebo effect is itself responsible for healing at least 30 percent of the time (Ref. #48, Chapters 1 and 12; Refs. #57 and #81). Healing from the placebo effect includes acne, arthritis, migraine, postoperative wound pain, and coronary artery bypass grafting. Furthermore the placebo effect spans physiological disorders to include altering emotional states and cognitive/mental processes. It is so powerful that the U.S. Food and Drug Administration requires that every new drug must be tested against a placebo to insure the drug's efficacy (Ref. #48, Chapter 1). Research on the placebo effect is itself further clinical evidence for the existence of psychoneuroimmunology.

The inert placebo effect just described is one type of placebo effect. It is the type most often thought of when a person is asked to describe the placebo effect. However, there are others. Four of these are :

- The active placebo effect
- The patient awareness of administered placebos
- The psychological factors eliciting the placebo effect
- The nocebo effect (Refs. #57, #81, and #95)

Active placebo effect. This is when a placebo has some specific physiological effect, though not for the intent of the treatment. For example, research has indicated that more than 90 percent of the patients reported improvement in their physical symptoms following coronary artery bypass grafting (diseased artery sections are bypassed/detoured via a new vein grafted from veins taken from the leg); and 75 percent of the patients performed better on stress tests. However, of these 90 percent, only 20 percent showed actual improvement of heart function when tested (Ref. #81). Another example is the prescription of antibiotics for virus-induced sore throats. Though antibiotics are made to counteract bacteria, many patients with this physical problem do experience rapid relief. Another incredible example of this effect: In a chemotherapy experiment, 30.8 percent of those patients who received placebos as a control group still lost their hair (Ref. #57)!

Patient awareness of administered placebos. The element of deception, the risk of losing their patient's trust, is a major reason why individual doctors will not use placebos. However, some patients do respond to placebos, even when told exactly what they are getting. In one study, 14 out-patient psychiatric clients suffering from somatic symptoms were told they were getting sugar pills to relieve their symptoms; 13 of the patients reported symptom reduction (Ref. #57).

Psychological factors. Psychological factors can also elicit the placebo effect. A common trait shared by all the above-cited research is the belief in the treatment and expectation of improvement held by either the healthcare provider and/or the client receiving the treatment. Thus confidence (belief) in the treatment and expectation are two psychological factors that apparently elicit the placebo effect. Other factors include:

- Meaning
- Manner, or process
- Message
- The physical characteristics of the treatment and its administration (Ref. #81)

Meaning. Ornstein and Sobel (Ref. #81) give an excellent example of this. A soldier wounded in battle experiences pain. A person injured in a car accident experiences pain. Perhaps pain in these examples means different things to the soldier than to the car accident victim. After a battle on a particular beachhead, only 25 percent of the soldiers needed pain medication for serious wounds. To the soldier, the wound was the ticket home. For the car accident victim, the accident meant more hassles with the insurance company, more hospital bills, lost work, etc.

Manner. What is the client's confidence level in the doctor prescribing the treatment? What is the doctor's in the patient? *Patient satisfaction* is defined as the response patients have toward their physicians based upon their perceptive of affective, behavioral, and cognitive components of the physician's behavior. Research results indicate patient satisfaction affects patient recovery. Satisfied patients are more likely to comply with treatment, which leads to recovery (Ref. #26). Doctor-client interaction in terms of their manner flows two ways. Patients who ask questions are perceived as motivated and taking more self-responsibility for their own care. Such patients motivate the healthcare team to supply them with more information, in turn, positively contributing to the doctor-patient trust and confidence (Ref. #96).

Message. What actual words are used? What words carry greater positive connotations? For example, is hair loss in chemotherapy presented as a possibility or as a certainty? What produces the self-fulfilling prophecy? Is chemotherapy presented as a powerful ally to the immune system or as a necessary, toxic procedure?

One research team reported on two groups of patients being given a placebo pill prior to injection of a pain suppression for dental work. But the verbal message differed for each group. One group's message was very confident in nature, with effects of the pill to take place almost immediately. The other group received a message to this effect concerning the pill: It reduces tension and sensitivity to pain in some people; other people receive no benefit. If it is going to work, it will work immediately. The healthcare professional also added that he personally had not found it to be effective (Ref. #81). The results: the group receiving the confident message experienced a significant reduction in anxiety and in pain perception.

Physical characteristics of the treatment and its administration. The following research results have been obtained in this category:

- Form apparently matters more than substance. There is a hierarchy of impact
- Placebo injections elicit a greater placebo effect than placebo pills; placebo capsules are less effective than injections but more effective than placebo pills
- Yellow placebo pills work well for depression
- Blue placebo pills have a greater impact if used as sedatives
- "More pain, more gain." The more a pill is bitter-tasting, the more unpleasant and/or difficult the treatment, the greater the placebo effect
- Brand names create a greater impact (Ref. #81)

Packaging the same placebo pill as a generic or as a nationally recognized brand does matter. The placebo packaged as the nationally recognized brand has more effect.

The nocebo effect. Just as a placebo is associated with a positive change, a nocebo (a negative placebo) is associated with negative change. This ties in with the psychological factors reported above. In the nocebo effect, the doctor gives a viable treatment that should work but the client doesn't respond physiologically to it because, psychologically, the doctor has signaled (verbally and/or non-verbally) that the drug isn't going to work. An example of this is the dental group's pain analgesic placebo pill, described above, under "Message". Dr. Naomi Remen has called this giving negative, false hope (Ref. #95). This negative hope may be given in verbal and/or nonverbal messages.

Spontaneous remissions. Medical research that advocates for the existence of the field of PNI also involves investigation of spontaneous remissions. This is the "nonscience of science" - perhaps an area medical science would like swept under the scientific Method rug. The still traditional medical view is that spontaneous remissions do not really happen. That the disease was misdiagnosed: The patient didn't really have the disease that went into remission; he/she had something else.

But something happened. The Institute of Noetic Sciences (Ref. #79) has assembled a data base of over 3000 articles in over 860 international medical journals. Twenty percent of their assembled data base deals with cures involving no medical intervention at all. Furthermore, this data base covers remissions from almost every disease known to traditional medical science. Any given article may deal with hundreds of known cases. Ref. #79 also documents some examples of the thoroughness of these reports.

Traditional medicine does not generally recognize "miracles" occurring through spiritual healing. However, 64 of the reported miracle healings in Lourdes, France (6000 claims from 1858 through 1986) have been officially declared miracles by the International Medical Commission. Their rigorous procedures and the commission member credentials are listed in Ref. #79.

Another type of spontaneous remission deals with multiple personalities exhibited primarily by people who have been severely abused (physically and/or sexually) as children. Multiple Personality Syndrome now accounts for one percent of all psychiatric cases (Ref. #75). As the personalities, termed alters in the field, change within the same body:

- An allergy present in one personality will disappear when another alter manifests
- Electroencephalograph (EEG) readings will reveal that brain wave activity will dramatically change from one personality to another
- Women may have as many as three menstrual periods in one month if three different female personalities manifest within that same month
- Some people will be allergic to a drug in one personality and not in another (Refs. #75 and #102)

Thus spontaneous remissions have been documented and studied, subject to the scrutiny of the scientific method. Such cases indicate an incredibly rapid, dynamic fluidity among the psyche, the body and its innate intelligence, and the body's healing systems.

Consequences and Applications

Research studies mentioned with the skills and disciplines of mind/body medicine within this book indicate that healthcare costs are reduced. This is in connection with disease and illness already diagnosed. The healthcare community could experience great cost savings if the medical community, including third party payers, and the general public incorporate mind/body medicine skills into wellness programming as an emphasis upon preventive medicine.

Considering the ever-increasing escalation of healthcare costs, already 16 percent of the total Gross Domestic Product, it is imperative that clients and practitioners alike begin implementing these skills into prescribed treatment - not as a substitute for traditional treatment but as a supplement to such treatment. Specifically, in regards to patient education, the roles outlined in Sections #3 and #4 become a means for such implementation.

More information on the skills and disciplines involved with psychoneuroimmunology are contained in various Sections throughout this book. The reader can also consult this book's resource section (Section #31) and Bibliography (Section #32).

References (Sources cited in this section): 26, 48, 57, 75, 79, 81, 95, 96, 102
References (Sources used as general reference works for this section): 1

#15: THE IMMUNE SYSTEM

Characteristics and Functions

The immune system is a complex network of billions of cells, hormones, and organs throughout the body which defend the body from disease. It, too, is part of mind/body intelligence. It, too, is fluid. For unlike the nervous system, whose cells are stationary, the cells of the immune system are highly mobile.

It is intelligent. It receives instruction and takes instructions from the brain. The immune system contains its own memory; it is capable of recognizing every toxin, bacterium, and virus existing in nature. It remembers how to fight viruses previously encountered and can instantly create new cells in innumerable combinations. Through vaccinations, inoculating a person with a mild form of a virus or bacterium for future protection, the immune system can be trained.

The immune system has three primary functions:

- To identify itself and what is naturally part of the body
- To identify what is foreign: not naturally part of the body
- To eliminate, destroy or render inactive what is foreign

In order to accomplish these tasks, the immune system has two major "arms" or "armies." These are:

- The humoral immune system (body fluid or semifluid, such as blood or lymph
- The cellular immune system (Ref. #48, Chapter 3)

The humoral immune system. In this subsystem, white blood cells called B-cells, or B-lymphocytes, produce *antibodies*. B cells circulate through the body's lymph fluid. The antibodies they produce are crucial in the body's defense against viruses and bacteria that invade the body through body fluids. These invaders are termed *antigens.*

The antibodies themselves are proteins, called *immunoglobulins*. Each antibody produced is programmed to attack a specific type of antigen, such as a flu strain virus, typhoid bacteria, etc. Using the lock and key analogy from Section #13, the antigen is caught by a B-cell surface receptor, having a molecular shape matching the antigen. The B-cell then engulfs the antigen, except for a portion of the antigen that the B-cell allows to be exposed on its (the B-cell's) surface.

This exposure attracts helper T-cells. These cells are sent from the thymus gland (hence their name) where they apparently are energized for action. Prior to this, they circulate through the lymph fluid. Thus, they are also a lymphocyte. A helper T-cell, attracted to the B-cell, will attach itself to the B-cell and release interleukins. These are chemicals that convert the B-cell into a plasma cell, which produces the antibodies (see above).

As it produces the antibodies (immunoglobulins), the plasma cell multiplies and the cells it produces, in turn, produce millions of antibodies that hunt down the antigen.

Antibodies render antigens harmless by:

- Neutralizing a virus by latching onto it - thus making it impossible to invade a healthy cell. A virus is an organism that can reproduce only by invading healthy cells and forcing the cells to create more viruses
- Latching onto toxins produced by bacteria, thus inactivating the toxins
- Coating the bacteria directly, which serves to bring in reinforcements in the form of other proteins or cells that destroy the bacteria

Helper T-cells use hormones called *lymphokines* to summon additional antibody reinforcers. One of these hormones, interleukin-1, causes fever, perhaps to "cook the enemy" by raising the body's temperature. Interleukin-1 is also produced by the brain, which further establishes the linkage between the brain and the immune system (Ref. #107).

The cellular immune system. This system fights viruses and other cells that have invaded healthy cells and live within that cell, thus infecting the cell. A virus or other invader controls the cell's machinery and forces it to make more of itself. The cellular immune system responds to foreign invaders not with antibodies but with various immune system cells. These are:

- Macrophages
- T-lymphocytes
- Cytotoxic (cell-killing) T-cells
- Natural killer (NK) cells

Macrophages (Greek: big eater) are cells constantly circulating through the body, engulfing and eating bacteria, viruses, and even dead cells. The engulfment occurs when a macrophage sends its cytoplasm flowing around the foreign particle and isolates it in a sac. The macrophage then shoots enzymes into the sac, destroying the substance and eventually itself. The body produces 100 million macrophages a day. This constitutes approximately 65 percent of the total white blood cell count.

Any cell that has been penetrated by a virus or cancer cell can signal for help. Bits of antigen protein will make their way to the surface of the cell.

Each natural cell contains a *major histocompatibility complex* (MHC) molecule. The MHC is an identity badge found on macrophages and other cells. It sees cells as friend or foe. Many researchers now regard the MHC as a linchpin of the immune system (Ref. #40). The MHC molecule will hold bits of the antigen for helper T-cells to recognize. Helper T-cells will help B-lymphocyte cells to produce antibodies.

T-lymphocytes, or T-cells, as a component of the cellular immune system, don't directly produce antibodies. They do attack foreign invaders (antigens) and help B-lymphocyte cells produce antibodies which are part of the family of proteins termed immunoglobins (see above). The term T-cell derives from the *t* in *thymus* gland, where much of the development of T-cells occurs (Ref. #48).

In the cellular immune system response, helper T-cells serve as the field commander of the immune system, calling in additional reinforcements. Two of these reinforcements are also in the T-lymphocyte group:

- Cytotoxic T-cells
- Natural killer (NK) cells

Cytotoxic T-cells constantly patrol the body searching for infected cells. Once they find them, these T-cells attach themselves to the infected cell and release packets of chemicals that destroy the cell. Like each antibody, each type of cytotoxic T-cell is designed and programmed to attack a specifically targeted antigen. Some attack cells infected by viruses; some attack cancer cells. A disadvantage of the cytotoxic T-cell is that some are programmed to attack transplanted organs and tissue which, up to the time of operation, would be "foreign" to the body's identification and memory of itself.

Natural killer (NK) cells also roam the body, searching out foreign cells. However, unlike the specifically targeted cytotoxic T-cell, each *NK* cell has a broad range of possible targets - from tumor cells to infectious microbes.

The Immune System and Memory

A key to the immune system's capacity for learning is another type of T-cell, called the *suppresser T-cell*. Again, helper T-cells stimulate the B-lymphocytes to produce antibodies and help activate other T-cells as above. The task of suppresser T-cells is to *shut down* the helper T-cells when enough antibodies have been produced. They serve a regulatory function (Ref. 48, Chapter 3).

At this time we do not know if these cells also function within the immune system's learning and memory "system" or the nature of such a system. Researchers believe in the existence of such a system, speculating that special T-cells and B-cells serve as memory cells that allow the body to remember how to counteract enemies previously fought (Ref. #40). This memory provides long-term immunity. It has been the basis for all vaccination programs since 1796, when Edward Jenner inoculated an eight-year-old boy with cowpox substance, which created an immunity in the boy when exposed to smallpox. His immune system was being trained to react and kill any foreign invader that resembled the cowpox virus, including smallpox virus.

Because the immune system can learn and remember, vaccination programs have become a great medical success story. Vaccines have been developed for such diseases as:

- Tetanus
- Smallpox
- Diptheria
- Measles
- Mumps
- Influenza strains
- Whooping cough
- Polio
- Chicken pox

The Overactive and Underactive Immune System

The health of the immune system is critical to the health of the body. One widely accepted theory is that cancer cells and some viruses like herpes circulate in the body constantly but are held in check by the immune system (Ref. #48, Chapter 3). These diseases can only take hold when genetic or environmental factors suppress the immune system's functioning. As Claude Bernard, considered the founder of experimental medicine, expressed it in the 1800's, the interior milieu is everything.

That is, research emphasis must be placed upon the body's internal ability to protect and defend itself against the external environment in which the body operates (Ref. #81).

AIDS (Acquired Immune Deficiency Syndrome) and cancer are major disasters to the immune system. Both suppress further an underactive immune system. AIDS patients have lower T-cell counts and excessive amounts of pathological antibodies. Given this immunological suppression, AIDS patients are unable to resist other infections (viruses and bacteria) and cancer (Ref. 48, Chapter 3).

An overactive immune system produces problems as well. Two major ones are:

- Allergies
- Autoimmune diseases

When the body's immune system becomes oversensitized to an environmental stimulus, it overreacts with an intense response, producing an allergic reaction. For example, hay fever is the result of the immune system's response to pollen in ragweed. Massive amounts of antibodies are produced: This in turn causes another type of white blood cell, *mast cells*, to produce histamine, a chemical which inflames the nasal passages. This in turn causes the symptoms of tearing eyes, itching, and sneezing.

At times, a person can go into anaphylactic shock - such as dying from a bee sting. In combating the poison, the immune system destroys the person.

Autoimmune diseases are another over reaction by the immune system. Such diseases occur when the immune system's cells somehow mistake the body's naturally healthy cells as foreign and it sets out to destroy them. Such autoimmune diseases include:

- SLE lupus (systemic lupus erythematosus)
- Multiple sclerosis
- Rheumatoid arthritis

Stress and the Immune System

Does stress (Section #17) cause disease? Research evidence to date indicates that it is difficult to clearly state that stress has caused a disease, in spite of the claims by many pop psychologists and holistic health practitioners that disease is dis-ease: "dis-easement". However medical research does clearly indicate that under long-term, chronic stress, immune system function is lowered (Ref. #48, Chapter

3; see particularly p. 51). Furthermore, people under stress actively pursue life style behaviors fostering stress, or "diseasement programming", rather than wellness programming, putting themselves at greater risk of incurring disease ("Wellness", Section #18).

Such life style behaviors involve:

- Alcohol and drug abuse
- Poor nutrition
- Physical inactivity
- Smoking
- Violent behavior

References: 40, 41, 48, 81, 107

#16: THE LIMBIC SYSTEM

Limbic (Latin): bordering or hemming in

Introduction

Recall from Section #15 that the immune system receives and takes instruction from the brain. A critical physiological component of the brain, for the purposes of this text, is the *limbic system* and the function it performs in relation to physical, mental and emotional health (Section #5). Prior to examining these functions, some background is necessary.

Beneath the cerebrum lies the mammalian brain, so termed because the same structure is found in all land mammals. This part of the brain most likely evolved 200 to 300 million years ago when the ancestors of homo sapiens evolved from the sea into a permanent land species.

The mammalian brain contains the limbic system. This system consists of two almost concentric rings, each connected to the cerebrum's left and right hemispheres (Section #9) and to each other via the hippocampal commissure (Section #9, Figure 9.2).

As mentioned in Section #13, the limbic system is rich in neuropeptides. Thus it is an integral component of the body's innate intelligence. It is part of the human brain; but within the brain's evolution, it has been a part of the mammalian brain.

The limbic system affects learning, physical health, and emotional health by performing three critical functions (Refs. #52, #56, #81, #82, #83, #103, and #112) :

- Physiological maintenance
- Emotional balance
- Learning and memory (transference of information into memory storage involving both short-term and long-term memory and its retrieval)

Physiological maintenance. The hypothalamus, a small gland about the size of a pea, is a part of the limbic system. The hypothalamus and limbic system together regulate (Refs. #52 and #81):

- Eating
- Drinking

- Waking
- Sleeping
- Body temperatures
- Hormonal balances
- Sexual drive
- Heart rate
- Blood pressure
- Blood sugar levels

Research has revealed that the hypothalamus is directly involved in the regulation of the immune system. It also directs the activity of the pituitary gland, which produces the chemicals and hormones that are carried throughout the body's cellular structure and are thus critical to the immune system and to health.

The two center rings of the limbic system enclose the thalamus; the thalamus is connected to the limbic system by a mass of nerves. The thalamus acts as the main relay station, analyzing stimuli and passing information (in the form of sensory impulses) through the nerves to other parts of the brain, including the neocortex.

These physiological functions of the limbic system help to maintain homeostasis, i.e., a stable environment for the body.

Emotional balance. In addition to acting as the physical thermostat, the limbic system also serves as the emotional thermostat and is often referred to as the emotional brain. In 1937, neuroanatomist James Papez of the National Institutes of Health postulated that the brain's neuroanatomical circuitry was involved in both thought and emotion. Subsequent electrochemical research validated Papez's theory and demonstrated that the limbic system helps to maintain emotional homeostasis of such paired emotions as (Ref. #52):

- Rage/fear
- Pleasure/pain (reward/punishment)
- Tension/relaxation (Section #10 - especially the "relaxed, yet alert" balance achieved with accelerated learning)
- Expectation/actuality
- Fight/flight response: without such balance, the human being would experience emotional extremes

Stress directly affects the limbic system, with the hypothalamus coordinating the physical and emotional responses to a stressor. (See also Section #17.) The limbic system, via the hypothalamus, readies the body to deal with a crisis (real or imagined) by stimulating the pituitary gland to secrete adrenocorticotropic hormone (ACTH). ACTH, in turn, triggers the adrenal cortex to pump adrenaline and to release chemicals that initiate the metabolism of proteins and fats into sugar, activities that provide the body with the energy and strength required for working through a crisis situation.

Additional physical reactions to a crisis include:

- Increased heart rate
- Elevated blood pressure
- Increased metabolic rate
- Muscle tension
- Release of blood clotting factors and enzymes
- Increased perspiration

These physical and chemical reactions literally pump the body up in response to a stressor, poising it for action. Such responses have enabled the human species to survive and evolve. Indeed, some researchers contend that the major purpose of the brain is survival and health maintenance (Ref. # 81).

In a complex society, crises may manifest themselves in less than concrete ways and create a fight or flight response that never shuts down. An animal's limbic system returns the body to physical and emotional homeostasis as soon as a threat is dealt with and/or removed. However, due to a sense of past, present and future time, man retains the memory of a crisis even after a stressor is physically removed from the environment or mentally removed from consciousness.

Man constantly collects and emotionally retains such experiences as rush hour traffic, job stresses, daily duties and major life crises, creating long-term, chronic stress. If left unchecked, this stress can lead to diseases, such as heart disease, which suppress the body's immune system (Section #15).

If the limbic system can produce the "fight or flight response", a reaction to a crisis as described above (also, Section #17), it can also produce "the relaxation response". It is the relaxation response that fosters physical healing. These benefits are described in Section #18.

Learning and memory. Learning is interconnected with man's ability to think. Learning can be defined as the registration of stimuli and their recall (memory) (Ref. #65). Some researchers do not distinguish between learning and memory, but they do differ.

Memory is the process of recall of data which has already been learned and encoded within the brain; thus, learning must precede recall. For the conscious mind, the recall of a memory involves two distinct processes (Ref. #65):

- The attempt to initiate a recall of any stored information. If successful, the attempt results in conscious recollection
- Conscious recognition that the memory (the information recalled) corresponds to the recall attempt

The limbic system aids learning and memory retention by serving two functions:

- Directing information, processed by the brain, into appropriate memory storage areas. These areas include the brain as well as other parts of the body
- Transferring information from short-term to long-term memory

The *hippocampus,* a component of the limbic system, has been discovered to play an important role in initial learning and short-term memory. Short-term memory consists of two types:

- Very short-term, lasting for a second or less. As the brain perceives information from the senses, it briefly retains the stimulus
- Short-term, lasting from several seconds to one minute. The capacity of human attention limits the amount of information a person can focus upon

Because the brain continually attempts to simplify the external environment, only a fraction of the information received is actually retained in memory. Very short-term memory works just long enough for the conscious mind to grasp information, after which information may be peripherally held for several seconds (but no longer than a minute) in short-term memory. Research has shown that the average individual can hold no more than seven to nine new items of information in short-term memory.

For information to be remembered, placed in long-term memory, it must be reinforced. Such reinforcement involves:

- Methods pertaining to a person's learning style(s) (Section #9)
- Imagery (Sections #11 and #26)
- Mnemonics (memory cues - Section #11; and Ref. #103).
- Format of material to be learned (Section #12)
- Music (Section #21)
- Relaxation (Sections #19 and #27)

Research indicates that memories, even sensory memories, are integrated in the limbic system (Ref. #73). For example, one component of the limbic system is the *rhinencephalon* (Greek: nose brain; also known as the hippocampus [Refs. #82 and #86]). The rhinencephalon is believed to be involved with the sense of smell. Certain smells evoke vivid imagery and associated memories (Section #11).

Consequences for Patient Education

Stress adversely impacts learning (Ref. #103). Certainly, a healthcare crisis is stressful. Thus learning is affected. These points have major ramifications for patient education and "teachable moments" (Section #10). By recalling the functions of the limbic system, by knowing the interrelationships of stress, relaxation, and learning, the patient educator can simultaneously foster both healing and learning.

References: 52, 56, 65, 73, 81, 82, 83, 86, 103, 112

CLINICAL HEALING SKILLS

Notes

#17: STRESS AND HEALTH

Stress and the Stress Response

The stress response (or cycle) is characterized in Figure 17.1. Stress directly impacts the limbic system (Section #16). The limbic system and the hypothalamus coordinate *the fight or flight response,* which is the physical and emotional response to a threat - real or perceived. The name for this response derives from the research of Walter Cannon, Harvard physiologist, at the turn of the twentieth century (Ref. #48, Chapters 1 and 14; and Ref. #81).

Table 17.1: STRESS

The positive
or negative
physiological response
(end result)
within one's body.
This response
is created
by
physical, mental and/or emotional
stimuli.
These stimuli
are in your
external (outside of your body)
and/or
internal (mind and/or body)
environment.
And these stimuli
interact with
your emotions.

The hypothalamus is the brain's brain. Together with the limbic system, it is involved in:

- Direction of the fight or flight response
- Regulation of various physical functions (see listing, Section #18)
- Emotional reactions (Section #16)
- Communication with the immune system (Section #15)

The limbic system, via the hypothalamus, prepares the body to deal with a crisis (again, real or imagined) by stimulating the pituitary gland to secrete ACTH. ACTH, in turn, triggers the adrenal glands (located on the top of each kidney) to pump adrenalin which contains the hormones epinephrine and norepinephrine, into the body. ACTH also releases chemicals that initiate the metabolism of proteins and fats into sugars. These activities provide the body with the energy and strength required to work through a crisis situation (Ref. #81).

The pituitary gland is the master gland of the body. This gland regulates the physical body through hormones such as ACTH. Hormones are chemicals manufactured in the brain and sent to targeted cells and organs of the body. The pituitary also triggers the release of endorphins (Section #13), natural pain killers, that may also help the body mobilize for the crisis by blocking the physiological and emotional sensations of pain.

Additional physical reactions to a crisis include (Ref. #48, Chapter 2):

- Increased heart rate
- Elevated blood pressure
- Increased metabolic rate
- Muscle tension
- Release of blood-clotting factors
- Release of enzymes
- Increased perspiration

These physical and chemical reactions literally pump the body up in response to a stressor, poising it for action. A *stressor* is defined as a factor perceived and experienced by the individual which produces stress (Ref. #98). Such responses have enabled the human species to survive and evolve. Indeed, some researchers contend that the major purposes of the brain are survival and health maintenance of the organism in which the brain is located (Ref. #81).

Thus, through the limbic system, the actual experiences, memories and the emotions related to those memories are interrelated. Hence the *interrelationship* of disease and illness (Section #5). This is why medical studies indicate that 70 percent or more of all visits made to a doctor are made by people with a

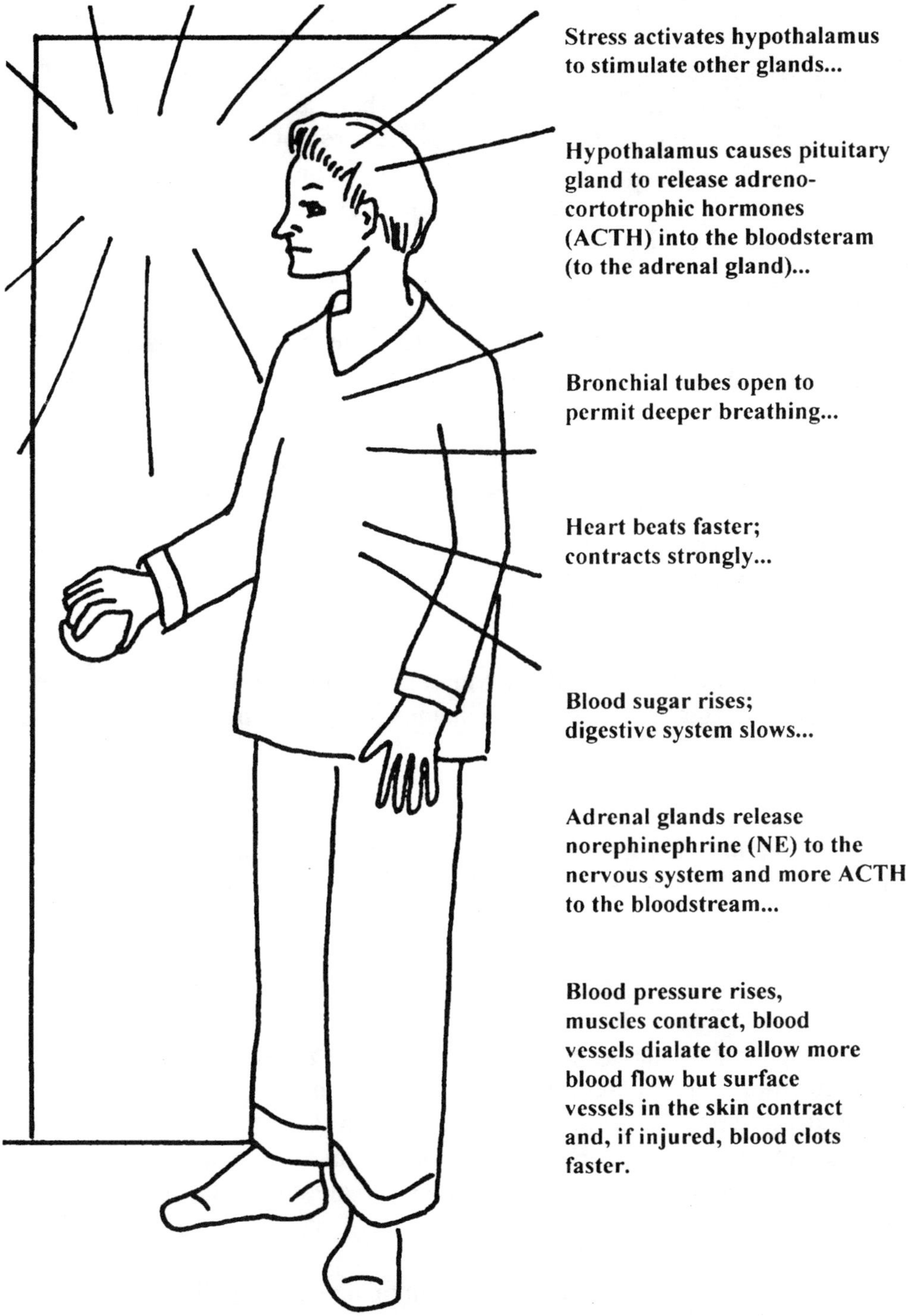

Figure 17.1. Reactions to Stress

stress-related disorder (Ref. #22).

These findings should not be interpreted by alternative healthcare practitioners or by the general public to mean that *dis-ease* is *disease*; that the state of mind or emotions or spirit will equal the state of the body. They are not the same, but they are related. Both illness and disease should be treated. Again, different levels of health are involved here (Section #5). Each level has knowledge bases, skills and resources commensurate with that level.

The reader must keep in mind that stress is a two-way street. Environmental factors, emotions and thoughts can aggravate disease. The disease itself is a stressor, creating stress which contributes to a person's emotional and mental state, affecting others in that person's environment.

Types of Stress

There are two major types of stress:

- Distress (from Latin: dis = "bad")
- Eustress (from Greek: eu = "good")

Distress is the negative type of stress. It is harmful and/or unpleasant, or perceived to be such. Distress, in turn, can be divided into two types:

- Episodic (short-term)
- Chronic (long-term)

Episodic stress and health. The above stress cycle depicts episodic, short-term stress and physiological changes. As the name suggests, the body is geared to face an immediate threat, real or imagined.

Chronic stress and health. If a person experiences chronic or long-term stress, the body continues to react. Due to the sense of past, present, and future time, a person retains the memory of a crisis even after a stressor is physically removed from the environment or mentally removed from consciousness. An animal's limbic system returns the body to physical and emotional homeostasis as soon as a threat is dealt with and/or removed. However, in our complex human society, crises may manifest themselves in less concrete ways and create a fight or flight response that never shuts down.

The body reacts to modern life as though it were still facing an immediate threat. People constantly collect and emotionally retain such experiences as rush hour traffic, job responsibilities and deadlines, and dealing with major life crises. The memory of the morning's rush hour traffic is fresh, along with all the emotions connected with it. The person thus directs the body to prepare itself for the impending crisis before the threat recurs. Thus the body is primed for the evening rush hour. The trigger/stressor is ongoing, throughout the work year, producing the ever-occuring stress cycle. This is an example of long-term, chronic stress.

Under long-term chronic stress, the initial physiological changes in the body produced by short-term stress are protracted, producing these results:

- Muscle tension can lead to headaches or aggravated pain
- Heart rate increases can lead to arrhythmia
- Blood pressure increases can lead to hypertension

Other physiological changes produced by chronic stress include:

- Loss of calcium from the bones
- An increase in blood cholesterol levels
- Suppression of immune system functions (Section #15), which in turn leads to increased susceptibility to bacterial infections, viral infections, and cancer

Hans Selye was a pioneer in stress research. In the 1950's, while at McGill University, he demonstrated that the body reacts to modern life stressors as if it were still facing an immediate physical threat. As Selye stated, the body's adaptability to stressors causing chronic stress is finite. Physiological change and disease do occur. (See also Section #19 and *eustress*, below.)

Chronic stress can produce more than physiological change. Other potential changes include the following categories and their specific symptoms (Ref. #48, Chapter 2).

- Cognitive changes:
    - Memory loss (Ref. #103)
    - Difficulty in ability to focus and concentrate
- Emotional changes:
    - Anxiety and worry
    - Feelings of hostility, irritability, and anger
    - Feelings of helplessness and hopelessness
    - Depression

- Behavioral changes:
    - Inability to sleep
    - Eating disorders
    - Increased reliance on drugs
- Social changes:
    - Increased sociability
    - Decreased sociability
    - Change in quality of relationships

Besides the physiological changes stress can directly cause, a review of medical studies listed in *Mind/Body Medicine* finds that stress aggravates these diseases (Ref. #48, Chapters 6, 7, 8, 9, and 11):

- Chronic pain. Patients believe that their pain is worse when they feel depressed and helpless
- Diabetes
- Skin diseases such as psoriasis, warts, and herpes
- Ulcers
- Gastrointestinal disorders
- Asthma

Stress also influences pregnancy (Ref. #48, Chapter 12). Pregnant women under major stress gain less weight because their metabolism is adversely affected by stress. The infant has a lower birth weight if the mother is experiencing major stress.

Eustress. Not all stress is negative. Seyle divided stress into *distress* and *eustress* (Ref. #98). Stressors (that which trigger the stress response or cycle) may be motivators. "Good stress" (eustress) may offer challenge and the opportunity for growth. A major function of the brain is to serve as the software for growth of the individual on all levels: physical, mental, emotional, and spiritual.

References: 22, 48, 81, 98, 103

#18: LIFE STYLE BEHAVIORAL CHANGES: STRESS MANAGEMENT AND WELLNESS PROGRAMMING

Overview

Two life style behavioral changes are needed to integrate the four levels of health discussed in Section #5, as well as the diverse skills and information found throughout this book. These are:

I. Stress management

II. Wellness

Both of these are considered separately, as subsections, within this section.

I. STRESS MANAGEMENT

Partnership Responsibility

Considering the consequences to health, stress management is a critical component in both the healing process and preventive medicine. Stress management works. We can never, nor should we, be free of stress. The overall goal of stress management should be reduction of distress and the creation of more eustress (Section #17). Both the healthcare provider and the co-therapist have joint responsibility in stress management.

The healthcare practitioner's responsibility, including the patient educator, is to make the client aware of the impact of distress and offer him/her skills and knowledge to reduce distress. The responsibility of the patient as partner or co-therapist is to acquire appropriate stress management skills and knowledge and practice them, incorporating them into his/her life as permanent life style behavior changes and a part of overall wellness programming (see below).

Components of a Stress Management Program: Consumer Tips

The reader should consult with his/her doctors and local hospitals to see if stress management education is offered. An appropriate resource person to talk to would be the patient educator or the hospital community affairs department. Outside the hospital, community resources include:

- County Mental Health/Mental Retardation workshops
- Wellness clinics
- Libraries

- YMCA and YWCA
- American Heart Association
- Local community colleges

An effective stress management program should have three basic components which will:

1. Help the participant identify individual stressors - including work and personal life stressors
2. Help the participant develop "stress hardiness" (see below)
3. Help the person practice the "relaxation response" (see below)

1. Identification of stressors. Various testing instruments are on the market to aid people in identification of individual stressors. A description of these instruments is beyond the parameters of this book. The reader should be aware that a comparison of an individual's composite score with a mean average is not an absolute prediction of physiological disease. Some early testing instruments provided a numerical composite stress score, based on a numerical scale assigned for each listed stressor, to predict the probability and time frame of disease occurring.

Research studies on such scales have not backed up their claim that a high stress level is commensurate with disease and/or other psychological problems. A predictor of disease is not a guarantee of disease. A statistic is just that - a statistic.

An effective testing instrument used in stress management programming is one in which the participant is helped to identify individual stressors - both personal and work related. This identification can help the participant know what type of skills are needed to reduce, if not eliminate, the impact of the stressor(s).

2. Hardiness. What research studies have also shown is that the nature of stress varies from individual to individual. Indeed, at times the major life changes are not the cause of breakdowns. The ongoing accumulation of small stressors is more likely to cause a breakdown..

Researchers believe that a component called *hardiness* is the key factor which enables one to adapt to stress.

Hardiness is defined as psychological strength. It consists of three major components:

- Control
- Commitment
- Challenge (Ref. #48, Chapters 2 and 81)

Control. There is a balance somewhere between control and controlling. The word *control* has both positive and negative connotations. As used in stress management, control means this: Are the resources at our disposal sufficient to deal with the stressor(s)? Distress occurs when our resources (time, community services, finances, friends, family, technological equipment, etc.) get outstripped by the demands imposed by the stressors.

A *controlling* person is usually aggressive: that person's rights come first. Others are simply possessions, without life or values. One verbal manifestation of the controlling person is overuse of the word *my: my* wife; *my* patients; *my* staff; etc. The word my implies ownership. "If I own 'it/them', they must adhere to the same values I do. I will spend my energy to see that they do." If they don't, stress and conflict occur. A controlling person usually ends up being possessed by his/her possessions and does not have the energy to keep up with everything. They do not take time to replenish their energy.

Commitment. To what values is the person committed? An effective stress management program will aid in values clarification. Commitment provides meaning in life.

Challenge. A stressor can be real, in actual concrete, empirical existence, or perceived. If I perceive that the stranger approaching me is going to mug me, I will trigger the fight or flight response. The perception that the person is a threat to me produces distress.

This concept of perception is critical for the upper right cognitive processor (Section #9). An upper right processor has a natural tendency to concentrate on the things that are going wrong, regardless of what and how much is going right. For this processor, the question is not whether the glass is half empty (pessimistic perception) or half full (optimistic perception); the question is: What is in the glass?

Or, the perceived squeaky wheel gets all the grease, regardless of whether or not it actually squeaks.

Do we fear/hate life or do we love life? Fear is the opposite of love, not hate.

Hate is a manifestation of fear. We do have control over our internal dialogues with ourselves. We do have control over how we perceive life events. Is the divorce a tragedy which I will never overcome or does it present me with a challenge? Are my immediate years ahead to be spent in fear of living alone or to be construed as an opportunity to learn from my mistakes, to learn my lessons, and move on?

Is a situation a threat or a challenge? Our perceptions of the situation may help dictate our answer to this question. Recall from Section #9 that a person with a "lower left" dominant cognitive thinking style is a low risk taker. This person also desires to have order and structure in his/her environment. Such a processor may be prone to view a situation as bereft with threats and not opportunity.

An effective stress management program will aid the participant in developing hardiness behavioral skills. Subject content can encompass a wide range, including any or all of, but not limited to, the following:

- Assertiveness training. There is a difference between assertiveness behavior (we both have innate rights as human beings) and aggressiveness (my rights come first; there is no room for negotiation)

  Effective assertiveness behavior is premised upon *self-centeredness* (centered in the self: *I* will decide who pushes my buttons and when, while respecting your rights.) Aggressiveness is based upon selfishness

  In training and counseling experience, without this value foundation of centeredness, long-term behavioral results are nil. The person after training may revert to hostile behavior, passive nonassertiveness, or passive aggressiveness

- Time management. Effective time management training will not turn the participant into an "efficiency nut", but rather help the person prioritize and clarify what is important

- Values clarification. This process has many different meanings, but one common component is the sorting out of one's own personal values from other values - cultural, familial, etc.

- Problem-solving and decision-making. Effective problem-solving and decision-making training will aid individuals in developing critical thinking

- Cognitive restructuring. Content can include the identification of irrational ideas underlying a situation, the basis for such internal dialogue, and skills to change the dialogues into more effective coping strategies. Rational emotive imagery is an excellent skill process to use in such training (Refs. #39, #59, and #64)

- Mind/Body behavioral medicine (psychoneuroimmunology) (Section #14) skills such as:
  - Hypnosis (Ref. #48, Chapter 16)
  - Meditation (Ref. #48, Chapters 14 and 15)
  - Yoga (Ref. #48, Chapter 14, and "The relaxation response")
  - Physical exercise (Section #28)
  - Nutrition (Section #29)
  - Humor (Ref. #27)
  - Relaxation (Section #19)
  - Biofeedback (Ref. #48, Chapter 18)
  - Music (Section #21)
  - Imagery (Sections #11 and #26)
  - Support groups (Section #24)
  - Environment (Sections #20 and #25)
  - Belief system (Section #23)

3. *The relaxation response.* The stress response is triggered within the body via the limbic system (Section #16). This response is described in Section #17. This emergency reaction, called the fight or flight response, is assisted by the *sympathetic* nervous system. Controlled by the brain, it takes over when action is needed, sending impulses/commands to the adrenal glands. When balance is needed and the body needs a return to normal, the *parasympathetic* nervous system takes over. It slows the body's heart rate and decreases body metabolism, for example. Both of these nervous systems make up the body's *autonomic* nervous system. Dr. Herbert Benson, a cardiologist exploring simpler methods to treat stress-induced high blood pressure, termed this response of the body to overstress (the fight-or-flight response) *the relaxation response* (Refs. #8 and #48, Chapter 14).

The autonomic nervous system is considered to be autonomous - not controlled by the mind. However, researchers have clearly demonstrated that a person can be trained to elicit the relaxation response as an antidote to stress (Ref. #48, Chapter 14).

The relaxation response is not sleep, but a state of being relaxed, yet alert. This resource is discussed in detail in Section #19.

Physical Benefits Derived from the Relaxation Response

Table 18.1 lists the physiological benefits derived from the practice of the relaxation response.

Table 18.1: PHYSIOLOGICAL CHANGES ASSOCIATED WITH THE RELAXATION RESPONSE ELICITED WITH DIFFERENT TECHNIQUES

Technique	Oxygen Consumption	Respiratory Rate	Heart Rate	Alpha Waves	Blood Pressure	Muscle Tension
Transcendental meditation	Decreases	Decreases	Decreases	Increase	Decreases*	Not measured
Zen and yoga	Decreases	Decreases	Decreases	Increase	Decreases*	Not measured
Autogenic training	Not measured	Decreases	Decreases	Increase	Inconclusive results	Decreases
Progressive relaxation	Not measured	Not measured	Not measured	Not measured	Inconclusive results	Decreases
Hypnosis with suggested deep measured relaxation	Decreases	Decreases	Decreases	Not measured	Inconclusive results	Not

* in patients with elevated blood pressure

Reprinted with permission from Consumer Reports Books.

The importance of an increase in alpha brain waves is as follows. At an alpha brain wave state, research has revealed:

- Relaxation increases

- Stress diminishes
- Ability for concentration and focus increase
- Healing increases
- Learning increases

(Characteristics and descriptions of all four brain wave patterns [alpha, beta, theta, and delta] are found in Ref. #103.)

The Mind/Body Medical Institute (Section #31, Resources: Mind/Body Medical Institute) has treated thousands of people. Its staff has produced many research results obtained with techniques that evoke the relaxation response. For example, in one research study using behavioral medicine interventions for chronic pain patients (Ref. #21), it was found that clients trained in behavioral medicine had a 36 percent reduction in clinic visits over a one-year period (traditional healthcare facilities). This 36 percent reduction for the first year equaled 511 fewer visits to a healthcare clinic. The same 36 percent reduction was retained over the second year. An HMO (Health Maintenance Organization) serving these enrollees performed a cost assessment of this program. Results found were:

1. A net cost savings of $12,000 of health costs was achieved for these patients during the first year they were enrolled in this chronic pain program.
2. $23,000 of net savings for these same patients was achieved in the second year of this program.

It must be emphasized that this is one specific program treating a specific ailment (chronic pain) for two years. But it would be interesting to speculate about the healthcare cost savings for thousands of patients over five years, for example, encompassing various ailments involving dozens of programs at dozens of hospitals.

The relaxation response has been used to (Ref. #48, Chapter 14):

- Reduce chronic stress, including psychological changes induced by anger, anxiety, hostility, depression and stress
- Treat hypertension
- Lower blood pressure in patients having hypertension by an average range of 5 to 10 millimeters of mercury (blood pressure is measured in millimeters of mercury)
- Treat symptoms related to cancer and AIDS treatment (as with the side effects of chemotherapy: nausea and vomiting)
- Treat chronic pain
- Treat cardiac arrhythmias

Behavioral Interventions Eliciting the Relaxation Response

The study mentioned above used the following behavioral medicine interventions:

- Elicitation of the relaxation response via breathing exercises (see Section #27) and relaxation tapes
- Knowledge of pain pathology
- Homework: assessing pain medication and side effects and keeping daily pain diaries in specific qualitative terms; alternating activity with rest
- Yoga
- Nutrition (Section #29)
- Cognitive restructuring involving communication skills and problem-solving

The reader will note from this discussion that behavioral medicine interventions are a *supplement* to traditional medical intervention and not a *substitute*.

Yoga is one of the methods found to elicit the relaxation response (Table 18.1). There are four major types of yoga found world wide. In the United States, the type suited to the predominantly Western Judeo-Christian culture is Hatha yoga: concentration upon breathing and the physical postures called *assanas*. (For a description of all four types of yoga, the reader is referred to Ref. #101).

The form of relaxation training known as *autogenic training* (listed in Table 18.1) was pioneered by Dr. Johannes Schultz in Germany. In this training, the focus is upon guided vocal cues to obtain feelings of warmth and heaviness in the limbs of the body. A detailed narrative for conducting this training is given in Ref. #22.

Progressive relaxation training as a form of relaxation was pioneered by American psychologist Edmund Jacobson in the 1920's. Here, the emphasis is on muscle relaxation. The therapy alternates between awareness of tension and relaxation, both consciously controlled by the practitioner (Detailed narratives for conducting and performing this type of training are given in Ref. #22.)

Another form of relaxation listed in Table 18.1, *zen*, is a form of Buddhism, one of the world's major religions. It is also a form of meditation.

Dr. Benson's research into ways of eliciting the relaxation response has involved years of studying the impact of prayer and meditation. Both invoke the relaxation response (Refs. #8 and #48, Chapters 14 and 15). All major religions have intrinsic esoteric skills, regardless of their dogmas. These skills may involve the years of studying the impact of prayer and meditation. Both invoke the relaxation response (Refs. #8 and #48, Chapters 14 and 15). All major religions have intrinsic esoteric skills, regardless of their dogmas. These skills may involve the repetition of a *mantra* (a repetitive sound or phrase, the purpose of which is to minimize interfering thoughts creeping into the mind), and gently refocusing upon the mantra when the mental distractions occur. (And they will. Swartz has spent over ten years in meditation training and practice.) Again, these skills are found in prayer and in meditative practices of all major religions. Allowing the co-therapist to use skills found within his/her religion is another way of creating the environment for the relaxation response to occur.

Regardless of the behavioral interventions used to invoke the relaxation response, skill development in practice of relaxation is a critical cornerstone to stress management programming.

Other Elements of Effective Stress Management

The stress management practitioner must model what is being taught. His/her training environment must be comfortable for the participant and reflect an environment conducive to both healing (Sections #20 and #25) and learning (Ref. #103).

II. WELLNESS

In Section #5, healing was defined as a movement towards wholeness. The authors define *wellness* as:

actively being in this movement towards wholeness.

Three fundamental characteristics of wellness flow from this definition:

- A movement towards wholeness
- An acceptance and appreciation of life
- A self-regulated healthcare system

A movement towards wholeness. In Section #5, the reader was presented with four levels (or components) of health: physical, mental, emotional and spiritual. Wellness is recognition of these four levels of health and taking advantage of the opportunity for growth in any one or more of these domains. Wellness is incorporation of growth-enhancing, health-promoting, permanent behavioral changes into one's life. It involves conscious awareness that these changes reflect *movement* and not fruition. Wellness involves an acceptance of our limitations as finite human beings while taking advantage of our opportunity to grow. As such, this movement towards wholeness seemingly implies a contradiction: "How can I be healthy if I am physically unable to be? How can I be sick and well at the same time? This doesn't make sense. Either I'm well or I'm sick. Get real."

These statements reflect Western culture's emphasis upon *duality:* either/or. Either I'm sick or I'm not. Either I have a job or I don't. Either this chair I'm sitting on is real or it is not. This sense of duality permeates our culture, which also emphasizes the materialistic physical domain. This permeates our healthcare system which emphasizes physical medicine. Even our psychological and religious counseling enters the domain of duality: Either I'm on the right path or I'm not.

This emphasis upon duality is not real or practical. It is unreal because it is not good science. In physics, a particle can be mass as well as a light wave at the same time. In mind/body medicine, the intelligence of the body converts thoughts into physical chemical action (Section #13). How can a thought without mass and space be mass and space? It is - given the research in the field of quantum physics.

Nor is emphasis upon duality and the physical realm good medicine. An emphasis upon physical health leads to the limitations of modern medicine (Section #6). The consumer may have feelings of hopelessness and helplessness, despair and depression, when the limitations and resources of modern medicine cannot counteract the finiteness of the human body.

The authors contend that a major reason underlying the healthcare practitioners' mental and emotional (even physical) detachment from the patient is their overemphasis upon the "physical cure or else" approach to treatment: "Why should I get attached to someone who is going to die?" For example, Swartz was a consultant to the oncology division of a major medical center on the eastern seaboard investigating the incorporation of wellness programming into the treatment program. When Swartz questioned the nurses about their perceptions of their functions, roles and responsibilities regarding wellness, 90 percent defined wellness as physical cure; their job was to physically heal their patients. This type of attitude leads to detachment from patients and contributes to stress, burnout, and turnover.

When wellness is defined as embracing the four levels of health, then staff attachment, yet detachment, become possible. One can be detached from the physical outcome of disease progression while attached to offering healing resources touching upon the other levels of health.

With this recognition of the four levels of health, what is real, what is practical, can be demonstrated in the example of a wounded healer. This person may be wracked with incurable cancer, yet mentally, emotionally, and spiritually be prepared for transition. Her affairs are in order after having, for example, reconciled with her estranged daughter. Atoning for past, self-inflicted guilt, arriving at peace with her God (however she defines God), she is ready. She is wounded physically but healed in the other dimensions of health. For her, there is no duality, no either/or. The duality dissolves. The way out is the way in, into herself and through herself. Wellness for her is dying well.

One valuable resource recently added to our healthcare system is Hospice (Appendix A). This organization is dedicated to the concept of dying well. There is no charge for its services and counseling. In some areas, if the patient is old enough for Medicare, round the clock nursing care is paid for to enable the patient to die at home. This organization believes that a person who is dying is still a person. The individual is to be made as physically comfortable as possible while maintaining his/her dignity, as he/she prepares to die.

The concept of the wounded healer is not uncommon in our healthcare system. Besides the example of Hospice, we have probably heard of such healers even if we have not directly experienced being in the presence of such individuals. This concept from traditional medicine comes close to what Asian religions mean about the unfolding of the lotus. It unfolds in many directions simultaneously. Each petal of the body represents many paths for growth, many paths to wholeness, while being delicate and beautiful, fragile and limited.

Acceptance and appreciation of life. The opposite of love is fear, not hate. Hate is a manifestation of fear. (See "Challenge," under "Components of a Stress Management Program", above.)

Wellness is an internal state of being, embracing all levels of health. As such, it embraces the continuum of health and disease. Components of me (physical, mental, emotional, and spiritual) can be unhealthy, while other parts of me can be healthy. I can be (and am) healthy and unhealthy at the same time. The either/or duality is dissolved, as seen in the example of the wounded healer.

Wellness is thus an internal state of being, of accepting and appreciating, not simply a state of doing or performing healthy behaviors (see below). Without this *being-ness*, our healthy activities become not the pursuit of a healthy life but running from the fear of death. For far too many people, the healthy life style becomes the pursuit of staying young. This is not embracing life, loving life, but rather fearing death.

If I love life, I must at least accept death. Otherwise, how can I understand, know, and appreciate life? Life and death are part of the same continuum. Though opposites, they are interrelated. I cannot appreciate health (for example, being free of pain) without experiencing "un-health": the experience of pain. Health and unhealth, though opposites, are an interrelated part of the same continuum. If wellness is wholeness as characterized above, I must embrace the whole. Wellness, then, is a state of being, in appreciation of the continuum of the human experience.

A self-regulated healthcare system. The first two characteristics of wellness described above serve as the value foundation underlying health-related activities and behaviors. The values provide intrinsic self-motivation for long-term use of healthy life style behaviors. Some of these health-promoting behaviors were summarized in the subsections "Hardiness" and "Behavioral interventions eliciting the relaxation response," in this section.

Effective wellness programming involves the adaptation of these skills into one's life. A systematic approach to managing one's wellness programming will involve skills and behaviors that relate to all levels or components of health: the physical (including nutrition, exercise and relaxation training); the mental (including cognitive restructuring and problem-solving); the emotional (including stress management skills); and the spiritual (including values clarification).

Differences Between Stress Management and Wellness Programming

These three characteristics of wellness programming are different from stress management programming. Wellness is proactive and growth-oriented. It encompasses all four levels of health. Many times, stress management has a reactive and very specific focus: elimination or reduction of stressors in one's life that create distress. Because wellness has as its foundation certain intrinsic values, it is self-motivating. With self-motivation, a person will tend to take responsibility for his/her own healthy life style changes that have long-term benefit. Stress management skills actually are one set of skills used within wellness programming to achieve life style behavioral changes.

References: 8, 21, 22, 27, 39, 48, 59, 64, 81, 101, 103

#19: RELAXATION

The Importance of Relaxation to Healing

As recalled from Section #16, in preparing the body to meet crisis situations, the limbic system causes the senses to be stimulated and the body poised for action. The physiological responses so brought about have been termed the *fight or flight response.*

These responses cannot be sustained on a long-term basis, however. Stress researcher Dr. Hans Seyle classified physical reactions to stress as the General Adaptation Syndrome (GAS). This is a three-stage phenomenon involving:
(1) Alarm reaction. This is a reaction to a perceived stressor in which the brain prepares the body by means of the fight or flight response.
(2) Resistance. This is an increased physiological response by the brain and body to the stressor.
(3) Exhaustion. In this stage, if the stressor is prolonged, such as in chronic, long-term stress:

- The body's store of energy and all energy reserves become depleted
- Resistance to the stressor decreases
- The probability of illness increases due to suppression of the immune system (Section #15 and Ref. #98)

Relaxation reduces stress and cuts the stress cycle. Recall from Section #18 that the relaxation response creates physiological responses different from the fight or flight response. These physiological responses include:

- A lowering of the rate of breathing
- A decrease in oxygen consumption
- A decrease in blood flow to the muscles
- An increase in blood flow to the skin and brain, producing sensations, feelings of warmth
- A shift in brain wave patterns from beta to alpha

Characteristics of an alpha brain wave state include the following:

- A reduction in stress
- An increase in relaxation
- Facilitation of healing
- Increase in mental alertness and concentration

Thus a relaxed, yet alert mental state is achieved in the alpha brain wave state (Ref. #103).

The physiological changes produced by the relaxation response are similar to those produced by *appropriate* music (Section #21). All relaxation methods are more effective when accompanied by the types of music and/or sound listed in Section #21. Furthermore, relaxation exercises are more effective when accompanied by imagery (Section #26).

Various types of mental concentration and skill development can elicit the relaxation response. These have been described in Section #18. Two relaxation exercises that Swartz has consistently found to be effective are listed with detailed instructions in Section #27.

The Relationship of Relaxation to Learning

The GAS process (described above) can be applied to overall performance as well as to bodily responses. As stress and anxiety increase, so initially does performance. After a period of time, however, performance - even basic learning - decreases because of exhaustion if the anxiety level continues to remain high or to increase. This principle comes into play whenever excessive stress and/or panic set in. For example, though they may be highly experienced, hunters or back packers can become lost in the woods and forget how to use their equipment when faced with particularly stressful situations.

The GAS process can also be applied to learning. As individuals concentrate intently for long periods, their learning becomes so stressful that they become less relaxed. Their learning performance ultimately declines.

Dr. Georgi Lozanov, the original pioneer of accelerated learning (Ref. #103), found that the opposite is also true. That is, learners have as much difficulty concentrating when they are profoundly relaxed as when they are profoundly stressed. In a too relaxed state, learners become drowsy and inattentive and their capacity for learning diminishes acutely.

As a means of avoiding this extreme, accelerated learning methods bring the learner to an optimal point of alertness - termed "relaxed, yet alert" - without undue stress (distress; see Section #17) and without inattentiveness. This relaxed, yet alert balance is evidenced as the alpha brain wave state described above.

A model applying accelerated learning to patient education has been presented in Section #10. Refer to Table 10.3: "Patient Education: a Teaching/Training Model".

References: 98, 103

TABLE 20.1
SHIFTING PARADIGMS OF THE CLINICAL HEALING ENVIRONMENT

The Present/Past:	The Emerging:
1. Healing = Physical cure.	1. Four levels of healing exist, with each level having its appropriate knowledge, skill, and values base.
2. Curing is done *to* patients.	2. Healing is done *with* patients.
3. A hospital is a large building housing technology and staff skilled in curing. Physical cure is the task to be performed.	3. Architectural design fosters healing. Form follows function. The function of a hospital is to accelerate the healing process on any of the 4 levels of health.
4. The focus is upon treating the specific disease and the body parts affected.	4. The focus is upon treating the whole person. Illness and disease are not the same.
5. Walls, sheets, and uniforms are white.	5. Color, art and designs promote healing.
6. Music has no role in cure.	6. Music (appropriate music and sound) fosters healing, including physical cure.
7. The patient is a patient.	7. The patient is a co-therapist.
8. The healthcare system is a car body and repair shop.	8. The healthcare system is a car body and repair shop as well as a driver instruction institute.

The authors acknowledge Komras and Associates (Section #31, Resources) for the format of this table as well as some of the general categories expressed within: paradigms 3 and 5.

#20: THE CLINICAL HEALING ENVIRONMENT

Overview

Table 20.1 reflects many of the themes, strategies and skills presented in this book. The clinical healing environment will mirror these tenets as well as reflect the home physical environment incorporated into Section #25. Research studies listed in each of the sections demonstrably prove that these skills and strategies foster physical cure as well as healing. (See Sections #14, #17, #18, #21, #23, #24, #25, #26, #28 and #29 for examples.)

Should the reader want further resources in this regard, he/she is urged to consult the Resources Section (Section #31) and inquire further from those organizations already implementing the emerging tenets listed in Table 20.1. As a good starting point, the authors recommend "The Art of Healing." This video is one segment of the Public Broadcasting System sponsored program, "Healing and the Mind with Bill Moyers" that was broadcast in early 1993 (Ref. #74). This particular video visits three hospitals and examines what each organization is doing to create a healing environment. (Refer to Section #31, Resources, for an address of this video series.)

Creating an environment for healing to take place is a great challenge for healthcare providers in hospitals today. Is it realistic? Some hospitals are able to truly practice patient-centered care. In the aforementioned Public Broadcasting System program, Mr. Moyers interviews the CEO of Mid-Columbian Hospital in Oregon. The hospital philosophy and morale was so positively patient-focused that it made a group of 20 nurses watching it together, co-author Peske included, very envious. How can it really work and what might be some of the areas where we should be able to make changes which would make the environment comfortable for people without sacrificing any quality?

Wondering if the hospital environment is created primarily for the staff and routine of departments, it is Peske's observation that nothing much occurs between Friday and Sunday. If any tests need to be done, they wait until Monday. A physician recently told Peske about a patient who needed further testing prior to discharge. He really didn't want her to leave the hospital before the procedure but she was anxious to go home. It was a Friday and the diagnostic test wouldn't be done until Monday. On Saturday, he decided to discharge her that day. His plan was to readmit her the following week if her pain continued and to reschedule the test. Again, for whose convenience is the hospital routine created?

In the not too distant past, hospitals were comforting, caring, nurturing places. Peske says that having her first baby was so enjoyable, although fatiguing, that she wanted to stay longer than four days. In the past, if hospitalization was indicated, most of us could go to the hospital and expect to be treated, to recuperate to the point of wellness, and then resume the normal routine. This is quite different from the way people generally now feel about hospitals.

Hospitals are hectic, stressful environments where people are diagnosed, treated, started on the road of recuperation, and then discharged to complete the recovery phase at home. Most of Peske's patients dread hospitalization. For people with chronic lung diseases, hospitalizations are feared, avoided, and denied. Readmissions are common for patients with lung diseases. The insidious onset of infection can creep up on the patient; and the patient can have a difficult time differentiating between the onset of infections and just having a bad day.

Peske believes strongly that she can teach her patients the signs and symptoms of infection; they can learn how to become detectives and determine if they are getting sick, aware of warning signs given by their bodies. She can help them help themselves to stay out of the hospital. This would be real cost containment. The patient will become a true partner in care.

Together we work at keeping the patient healthy. If we are to truly establish clinical healing environments, we need to recognize the patient as a physical, emotional, mental, and spiritual being: a whole person.

What do you see in your environment that makes you comfortable? How does it affect your body and mind? What is your favorite imaginary scene? In your mind, where would you rather be now? What are you picturing? What kind of music relaxes you? When you visit art galleries or are at home, what effect does your favorite painting have on you?

Although it might seem radical, people who work in traditional healthcare environments need to consider the things that have positive, healing effects. Such consideration will help us create healing environments for our patients. We need to know about the effect the following have on us and our patients:

- Posters/artwork
- Colors (Section #25)

- Music
- Lighting (see "Environment in the waiting room", below)

For more information on this topic, see Sections: #19, Relaxation; #21, Music; and #26, Imagery and Healing, respectively.

When we know the effect of environmental stimuli on healing, we can use this to the best advantage to help create an environment where our patients can experience mental, emotional, and spiritual healing, as well as physical healing.

The following paragraphs give some specific examples of what a hospital clinic and/or its staff can do. They are not meant to be all-inclusive.

The Healing Environment of the Elderly

Dr. Creditor (Ref. #30) studied the impact of hospitalization upon elderly (age 75 or above) patients. Regardless of the condition for which they are admitted, elderly patients suffer the following as a result of a few days of bed rest:

- Loss of muscle strength. This loss of muscle strength due to bed rest, combined with a bed design that may include high bed rails, contributes to falls by the elderly
- Reaction to medical devices. Devices such as oxygen lines, intravenous lines, and catheters can become restraints, increasing the perception of the need to void waste, and leading in turn to urinary incontinence
- Sensory deprivation: Elderly patients can suffer delirium as a result of sensory deprivation. This can be caused by: glasses and/or hearing aids left at home, the hospital room environment, with a lack of clocks, calendars, and colors; the unfamiliar hospital diet; subdued lighting; eating in bed with trays, water, utensils that are difficult to reach; deprivation of reality orientation, such as daily dressing and undressing; and a lack of newspapers and magazines

Dr. Creditor states that these patients are not injured in falls out of bed but in trying to climb out of a high bed. He recommends new types of beds available on the market as well as easily cleaned carpeting that would provide a safe footing.

Dr. Creditor cites research which shows that the elderly patient suffers negative impact from hospitalization within the first two days. Yet the hospital geriatric assessment team, among whose functions it is to identify risk factors for that patient, usually doesn't meet until several days after the elderly patient is admitted.

By then the damage has been done; and the team recommendations have yet to be made.

These problems contribute to the elderly being shuttled to a nursing home that typically lacks the resources to rehabilitate the patient back to a pre-hospitalization functional level. One study cited by Dr. Creditor indicated that only 12 percent of such patients (originally hospitalized and subsequently referred to nursing homes) were eventually discharged to their home.

Waiting Areas for the Caregiver

Although much credence is given to the need for quality social support from the care giver, the hospital environment seems to do all it can to avoid such support. Most readers can recall memories of waiting room experiences that attest to the truth of this statement.

The "waiting room" environment could contribute to stress management in the same way as the home healing environment described in Section #25. The ideal hospital waiting area would include these features:

- Visiting hours are replaced by accessibility for overnight stays
- The patient and the caregiver both have access to the charts
- Children have accessibility to a game room that has hand and finger puppets, teddy bears, story books, etc. Parents are encouraged to bring in a child's favorite "warm fuzzy" from home
- Accessibility to a kitchenette
- Reading material encompassing general patient education material through humor and current periodicals
- Facilities for playing environmental videos and/or musical cassettes (See "Appropriate music" in Section #21). Ear phones are available and volunteers can instruct in equipment use
- Accessibility to an area where one can lie down and rest
- Accessibility to the following staff or a house phone that lists numbers for:

    Patients Rights advocate
    Patient education coordinator
    Chaplains
    Volunteers as needed (such as a clown)

- Accessibility to staff who, during a long surgical procedure, could inform the caregiver as to procedures progress, events, etc.
- A natural environment containing:

- Environmental posters if windows do not overlook a natural environment
- Full spectrum lighting (see Lighting, Section #25)
- Comfortable chairs
- Comfortable writing surface
- Earth tone colors with accents of salmons, mauves, yellows, etc. (Section #15)
- Plants, preferably natural, but artificial also provide a comforting touch

The authors advocate the position of patient advocate, who could help ensure that environmental considerations are made part of the healing environment for both the patient and the caregiver.

References: 30, 74

#21: MUSIC

Definitions

Sound is defined as mechanical radiant energy that is transmitted by longitudinal pressure waves and is perceived by the sense of hearing. Pressure waves are measured in decibels, the units used to express the relative loudness of sounds. One decibel equals approximately the smallest degree of difference of loudness ordinarily detectable by the human ear. The range of the human ear includes about 130 decibels on a scale for which one decibel correlates with the faintest audible sound.

Noise, though it is usually noticeably loud, harsh, or discordant, is defined as sound that lacks agreeable quality, regardless of its volume. As unwanted sound, it is a psychological as well as a physical phenomenon.

Music is the combination and organization of vocal or instrumental sounds possessing harmony, rhythm, and melody to produce a unified composition having structure and continuity. Described as agreeable sound, music is often referred to as the language of the emotions.

Physiological Impacts of Sound

Research has indicated that hypertension, often associated with high levels of stress, is increased by loud and sustained noise and that long-term exposure to sound above 90 decibels can result in hearing loss. Some examples of everyday sounds and their decibel levels/ranges are (Ref. #50):

· Live rock music, amplified	90 to 130
· A screaming child	90 to 115
· An alarm clock	80
· A dripping faucet	40
· Rush hour traffic	75 to 85
· A power lawn mower	100 to 105
· Vacuum cleaner	70 to 75

Physiological Impacts of Music

Like stress, music impacts the body both positively and negatively (Sections #17 and #18). Because instrumental music is nonverbal, it moves directly through the brain's auditory cortex to the limbic system (the center of emotional responses [Section #16], where it induces the release into the body of endorphins (opiate-like chemicals that relieve pain and produce euphoric feelings).

Music also impacts (Refs. #15 and #82):

- The heart, which normally beats between 70 and 80 times per minute but adjusts to synchronize with music tempos
- The respiratory rate, which synchronizes with music tempos
- Blood pressure
- Stomach contractions
- Levels of stress hormones in the blood (high levels appear to suppress the immune system)
- Physical reactions to stress:
    - Fast tempos generally heighten arousal
    - Slow tempos generally help lower physical reactions to stress
    - Brain wave rhythms synchronize with musical tempos

    One study demonstrated that, at 60 beats per minute, all four brain waves become proportionately balanced. Lozanov, the Bulgarian psychotherapist considered the father of accelerated learning (Ref. #103), discovered that music with 60 beats per minute, particularly Baroque classical music, facilitated accelerated learning.

Positive Impacts Upon Healing

Ornstein and Sobel (Ref. #82) reviewed research literature and found that:

- Classical music played before, during and after surgery:
    - Reduces patients' anxiety
    - Reduces patients' pain
    - Reduces the need for preoperative and postoperative medication
    - Accelerates healing
- Combined with Lamaze birthing methods, appropriate music reduces the duration of labor by as much as two hours
- Music is often used in the treatment of patients whose illnesses involve strong emotional components

Such evidence, combined with the fact of interactions between the mind and body, suggests that illness should be treated holistically. For every disease there are physiological and psychological components, the former being the natural organic progression of disease and the latter being the emotional "dis-ease" (stress and anxiety) of the patient. Correctly used, music can enhance the healing of both the disease and the related illness.

Because of their awareness of the impact of music, many physicians play Baroque music while performing surgery. Even plants have been proven to grow especially quickly and to remain in excellent health in an environment of classical music.

Music as medicine cuts across all healthcare disciplines. Considering the evidence, it seems logical to include its use in the fostering of environments conducive to healing whenever possible.

Negative Impacts Upon Healing

The negative consequences of music are as emphatic as the positive. Plants, for example, wither in the environment of rock music (which can range from 90 to 130 decibels). Some patients have been found to be addicted to music. Halpern (Ref. #50) asserts that sound and rhythm can be as addictive as any known drug; and Tame (Ref. #104) interviewed rock musicians who believe that they can create audience hysteria at will through their music.

Tame also cites 76 documented cases of musiogenic epilepsy (Ref. #104), a condition in which music causes seizures. Halpern cites the results of a major study, which reveals that when rock music is played during physical exercise, 90 percent of the participants lose strength and muscle coordination (Ref. #50).

Shrill sounds projected into liquid protein have been found to coagulate the protein. Tame cites experiments in which a raw egg placed on stage during a rock concert has cooked to a hardened state by the end of the concert. Swartz contends that the greatest negative effects come not from the lyrics (such as in rock music) but from the high volumes, fast rhythms and disharmonies of the music. These characteristics reinforce violent behavior because of their associative appeal and their appeal to the emotions, thus helping to create an environment that is very different from one conducive to healing. (See "Environmental sounds," below; and Section #25, "Natural environment".)

How Music Facilitates Learning

Various research studies indicate that the proper use of music facilitates and accelerates learning and health (Ref. #15).

Music directly affects the limbic system (Section #16). Recall that one of the three primary functions of the limbic system is that of information processing, storage, and retrieval. Music also appeals to the emotions, another limbic system function, and is known to be strongly associative, evoking imagery (Sections #11 and #26).

The limbic system is interconnected by the hippocampal commissure and physiologically connected with the right and left brain hemispheres (Section #9). The right and left brain hemispheres are connected by the corpus callosum. Music facilitates and supplements these natural interconnections, assisting the cerebral hemispheres and the limbic system in coordinating their functions, in working together in harmony.

Music also facilitates the creation of alpha brain waves, a pattern which aids in stress reduction and enhanced learning. (For a listing of the characteristics of alpha brain waves, refer to Section #18.)

Appropriate Types of Music and Sound

The three types of music and sound that facilitate both learning and healing are:

- Classical music
- Alternative music
- Environmental sounds

Classical music. Learning is facilitated when accompanied by Baroque and other classical musical selections having *andante* (moderately slow; a quarter note tempo of 40 to 72 beats per minute), *adagio* (slower than andante; a quarter note tempo of 50-76 beats per minute), and *largo* (slower than adagio; a quarter note tempo of 42 to 66 beats per minute) tempos. Authorities differ on the exact number of quarter note beats per minute of these tempos. However, one metronome lists them as follows: largo, 40 to 60 beats per minute; larghetto, 60-66; adagio, 66-76; and andante, 108. These tempos approximate the 60-beats-per-minute range that enhances accelerated learning.

Researchers of accelerated learning methods have discovered that, although the physiological state produced in participants listening to classical music of the 60-beats-per-minute range was unlike meditation, the physiological effects were similar to those produced by meditation, including:

- Lowered blood pressure

- Reduced breathing rates
- Reduced heart rates

The participants were relaxed, yet alert, and were able to focus and concentrate. Their electroencephalograph (EEG) brain wave patterns displayed an increase in alpha (associated with alertness) and a decrease in delta and theta (associated with drowsiness) brain wave patterns (Ref. #84).

These same participants, in spite of their intense mental activity, also displayed an overall decrease of beta brain waves, a pattern often associated with states of anxiety and prominent in the appropriate brain hemisphere involved with the mental task at hand.

Composers spanning the Baroque period of classical music (approximately 1600-1750, including J.S. Bach, Scarlatti, Handel, Haydn, Vivaldi, Corelli, Pachelbel) did not write song titles as we would term them today. Rather, their titles were the signature: the names of the tempos were instructions to the conductor as to how fast to play the composition:

largo: very slow
adagio: quite slow
andante: a walking pace

When you, the reader, select this type of music for purchase, look for these song titles. They will be listed. See "Positive impacts upon healing," above, for information on the impact of classical music upon health.

Alternative music. Alternative music (at times in the past it has been known as New Age music) is a growing segment of the recording industry, with radio stations across the country devoting programs to this type of music. No specific definition of this genre has been determined; even composers and musicians of the genre cannot agree on a definition. However, there are a few common characteristics that music of this type seems to share:

- It is primarily nonverbal and is designed to be as unobtrusive to the listener as possible
- The musical rhythms contained in this music are not *stopped-anapestic*; i.e., there is no beginning, middle, or end. Much popular music contains this stopped-anapestic rhythm, which consists of a short-short-long-pause pattern. This pattern was the one found associated with the physical workout research study cited by Halpern (Ref. #50)
- Alternative music is designed to foster a state of relaxation, enabling the listener to transcend time and space (via the right hemisphere's function of timelessness; see Section #9 for a listing of brain hemisphere functions)

- Alternative music compositions approximate the 60 beats per minute tempo
- This music is cross-cultural, reinforcing the quality of transcendence (transcending time and space) by utilizing instruments of various cultures
- Musical compositions often incorporate synthesized special effects with instrumental and environmental sounds

Appendix C lists selections containing these characteristics.

Environmental Sounds

An overwhelming majority of participants in Swartz's training programs find themselves imaging outdoor locations when they are asked to create a relaxation sanctuary (Section #27), with some indicating that although they consciously selected an indoor site, they found themselves mentally outdoors. Additionally, most report an association with water, regardless of the indoor or outdoor location.

This is no accident. The body, naturally relaxed, vibrates at a rate of approximately 7.8 to 8 cycles per second, approximating the rate of the brain's alpha brain wave state (Ref. #103). Geophysicists have demonstrated that the earth vibrates at this same frequency (Ref. #50). Human beings automatically become attuned to nature and its harmonies when in a relaxed state.

Research has concluded that a state of relaxation is promoted by environmental sounds, such as:

- The ocean surf and sea gulls
- A trickling stream
- Birds singing
- Crickets chirping
- The environment of a tropical rain forest

The authors recommend creating and maintaining a state of relaxation by playing either classical or alternative music simultaneously with an environmental sound tape that is associated with one's created relaxation sanctuary (Section #27).

Additional Musical Notes

The end of the '80s and the beginning of the '90s have seen two musical camps emerging as music is being applied to the fields of education and training. Those in one camp advocate the strict application of classical music for learning enhancement; those in the other advocate alternative music because it has the advantage of promoting relaxation without focusing upon the familiarity of much of classical music. It must be noted, however, that the popularization of alternative musical compositions will eventually lead to the familiarity argument being raised against the latter type of music as well.

The authors feel the greatest learning enhancement may come from the use of *both* music types, supplemented with recordings of environmental sounds. Healthcare professionals do a disservice to clients, staff, and patients if they allow stress management/wellness consultants to omit the use of appropriate music as a part of such program services as:

- Learning and training methodology
- Relaxation skills development
- Training workshop subject content
- Technical assistance services

Healthcare professionals also deprive themselves if they do not incorporate "sound nutrition" into their own health maintenance and wellness programming as well as their own learning and study processes. See Refs. #84 and #103 as well as Section #31 for resource information regarding the effective use of music in accelerated learning.

Finally, it is critically important to keep this point in mind:

**The mind may like hard rock and other music of this ilk,
but the body doesn't.**

Healing and learning are facilitated with the types of music presented in this section. As of 1993, the newly created Office of Alternative Medicine, National Institutes of Health, funded thirty research projects to further ascertain the power of music upon healing. It would be good if all researchers kept this critical point in mind when developing the methodologies for their studies.

References: 15, 50, 82, 84, 103, 104

#22: COMMUNICATION SKILLS

Overview

Communication is a process of information exchange. It is basic to understanding another person and is intimidating and/or stressful at times. Communication can be both verbal and nonverbal and is always time and space related.

Verbal communication is based on understanding language. Words are the essence of language. Words come from the cerebral processes involving the brain's left hemisphere (Section #9). Words have meaning in the particular language of the culture of the person speaking them.

Communication transcends all body functions. It subsumes the whole body: physical, mental, spiritual, and emotional. Holistic healthcare utilizes the total mind/body relationship in caring, nurturing and teaching patients. The holistic approach to healthcare (see traditional/alternative medicine sections) is a process of communicating with people.

The art of medicine and nursing practices techniques of communication involving the senses. On the conscious levels, these are:

- Seeing
- Hearing
- Touching
- Smelling
- Tasting
- Motion

(For all levels of senses, see Section #26.)

Some experts feel that the art of medicine and nursing has been lost. Some patients would agree that the soft, subjective art of healing has been lost, never to be regained. The public perception that it has been replaced by cold, calculating scientific data -solely - is not far from the truth. Pertinent questions for healthcare providers with respect to short-term and long-term communication are:

- Have our patients lost their sense of trust and confidence in us?
- Is the fast-paced time in which we live affecting our communication skills with our patients?
- How can we regain the sense of trust, confidence and commitment our

patients expect and need?

Hamlin (Ref. #51) states that approximately 15 percent of the brain is engaged in processing and in understanding verbal communication. This leaves approximately 85 percent of the brain's cognitive processing function that can be devoted to both verbal and nonverbal communication.

The realities of the time-pressured, physically and emotionally demanding hospital environment may sometimes prevent healthcare providers from truly listening. When barriers to listening exist, no communication can take place.

Verbal communication depends upon effective use of language. Positive outcomes for patients are based on principles of effective communication. Discovering what the patient is communicating verbally and nonverbally requires astute interviewing skills on the part of the healthcare provider. For example, older patients often answer questions with rambling answers. It is important that the healthcare provider learn how to:

- Focus the conversation
- Redirect the conversation when necessary to the problem at hand
- Ask visitors to step outside the room, if necessary
- Use only a few minutes at a time
- Be flexible if the patient is not able to listen due to discomfort

Healthcare practitioners who provide information to patients through patient teaching also need to be aware of the impact of nonverbal communication on patients. Patients show by their grimaces, tense fists, tense shoulders, and tightened jaws that they are uncomfortable. Healthcare providers display impatience and other nonverbal judgments (such as avoidance of eye contact) when they are uncomfortable due to the overwhelming number of tasks to be performed which reduce needed time with patients.

Truly listening to, and showing concern for, a patient is a risk. However, a mutual trust will only grow when healthcare providers are truly honest with patients. In the teaching/learning process, honest communication is vital to the success and effectiveness of learning. Honest communication only occurs when the healthcare provider and the patient experience a point of connection. This point between patient and healthcare provider or learner and teacher is called the *teaching connection.* Only at this point of mutual trust and understanding can effective patient education occur.

What Communication?

Doctors constitute one of the two primary, critical contacts a patient has with the healthcare system. Nurses represent the other, simply because of their direct contact with the patient (Ref. #88). Nurses also are the greatest resource for implementing patient education (Ref. #93).

Yet as Dr. T. Ferguson states (Ref. #48, Chapter 25), "bedside manners" of physicians are atrocious. Ferguson reports that the general practitioner spends an average of seven minutes with a patient. Of this time, most is spent in talking, not listening.

Roter and Hall (Ref. #96) state that according to most estimates, the length of the primary care medical visit in the United States lasts less than 20 minutes, while the average family practice visit is approximately 14 minutes. This includes:

- Periods of silence between patient and doctor
- Interruptions for the doctor
- Review of notes from a prior visit
- Several minutes of note taking at the end of the session

Roter and Hall (Ref. #96) conducted research regarding patient-doctor communication. Some of their conclusions follow:

- The physician's opening question to the patient was allowed to be fully answered by the patient in only 23 percent of the visits
- In 69 percent of the office visits, the physician interrupted whatever the patient was saying after a 15 second response by the patient
- Half of the physician talk time consists of giving facts. If physicians ask questions, they usually ask close-ended questions (See "Communication skills: questioning", below)
- Patients use only 6 percent of the time of a typical office visit to ask questions
- Patients seen earlier in the day have longer office visits than those seen in the afternoon
- Emotions and feelings are seldom addressed by patient or physician
- Research studies consistently indicate that patients want information related to diagnosis, disease origination, and prognosis. Consistently, doctors underestimate these needs and overestimate the importance placed upon treatment issues by the patients, particularly drug therapy
- Health means different things. For the doctor, health means absence of disease. For the patient, health includes functional abilities related to

quality of life issues and emotional distress as well as medical condition

In a 1993 research article in the New England Journal of Medicine (Ref. #38) regarding the use of unconventional alternative medicine and therapies, the authors state that more than 70 percent of those using such therapies do not tell their doctors about this use.

In a 1991 American Medical Association survey cited in Ref. #48, 58 percent of the respondents stated that doctors don't explain things well to their patients; 69 percent stated that most doctors don't spend enough time with patients.

Redman (Ref. #93) cites several nursing research studies with these findings:

- Too much information is withheld from patients
- Not enough time is available to teach patients
- Patients do not have enough knowledge to care for themselves after discharge
- Only 50 percent of patients surveyed were able to recall receiving education
- Nurses spend twice as much time educating as physicians

There may be several reasons for this lack of communication. Among them are:

- Barriers to patient education (Sec. #1)
- Physicians receive little training, if any, in communication skills during their medical training (Ref. #60)
- Physicians are paid, via third party payers, to make diagnoses, not to counsel
- Third party payers give little attention to the provision of patient education services

Patients may have difficulty in communication because they:

- May be conditioned to nonassertively accept traditional authority and power (skills and knowledge of the doctor)
- May be in denial as to the reality of the disease
- May trust an alternative medicine practitioner or therapist more than the medical doctor (Sec. #7)
- May be experiencing so much stress and anxiety due to both disease and illness that information is quickly forgotten. (Stress impedes learning and long-term memory retention [Ref. #103])

The Importance of Communication - Verbal and Nonverbal

Communication is vital. Lack of communication is certainly potentially harmful to one's health. Effective communication, including patient education, enhances the quality of care, increases compliance with treatment, and fosters cost containment. Burgoon, Birk, and Hall (Ref. #16) report that noncompliance with drug regimens is from 46 percent to 62 percent; medical appointment keeping noncompliance is 50 percent; and noncompliance with oral chemotherapy treatment is 59 percent. The latter point (cost containment) is covered in more detail in Section #2. With regard to the first two points, (quality of care and treatment compliance), Conlee, Olvera, and Vagim (Ref. #26) have surveyed research studies pertaining to the subject of communication. Their analysis of the literature (including references) indicates the following:

- Effective reciprocal communication (understanding) in the physician-patient relationship is an important predictor of recovery
- Satisfied patients may be more likely to comply with prescribed treatment (However, another review by the authors of the sources cited by Conlee, Olvera and Vagim in Ref. #26 indicates that the research is mixed on this point; there is no clear consensus)
- Patient compliance with treatment, including advice and information provided, directly and positively relates to recovery

What constitutes patient satisfaction with their doctors? Conlee, Olvera, and Vagim (Ref. #26) report that satisfaction was fostered by communication skills involved with the following factors:

- Respect/Attention. Verbal communication attributes involve these statements: "My physician listens to me." "He/she really tells me all aspects of my disease." "He/she treats me as a whole person, not just a physical body"
- Competence. Verbal or written communication attributes relate to a physician giving or not giving a patient information, such as drug side effects
- Humility. Verbal communication attributes relate to: being able to tell the patient when he/she has made a mistake; being able to refer to another specialist if the physician feels he/she cannot help the patient
- Accessibility. Communication attributes revolve around issues of availability and logistics: "Can I see my doctor in the evenings?" "On weekends?"

Conlee, Olevera and Vagim report (Ref. #26) that nonverbal communication also impacts patient satisfaction. (See also the impact of the placebo and nocebo effects reported in Section #14.) Their own research indicates that nonverbal communication attributes are included in the above-identified four factors constituting patient satisfaction. Nonverbal factors include:

- Eye contact
- Tone of voice
- Appropriate touch
- Space and distance: close, but appropriate social distance apart
- Positive head nods
- Smiles
- Body orientation to patient
- Nonverbal gestures connoting and conveying relaxation

Burgoon, Pfau, et al (Ref. #17) report that patients are more likely to be satisfied with their doctors when their verbal and nonverbal communication is perceived by the patient as displaying the following qualities:

- Openness
- Interest
- A willingness to listen
- Warmth
- Active involvement in my problems, a sense of equality, and a sense of formality (conveying expertise, knowledge, and authority)
  (The reader is encouraged to refer to Section #1 with respect to how the compensatory model for coping and helping aids in establishing a sense of equality.)

Roter and Hall (Ref. #96) cite two studies that find a positive relationship between doctor-patient conversation and patient health status. (They also cite numerous studies on communication that involve patient education, counseling, and behavioral medicine techniques.) In one study, patient blood pressure improved when the patients were allowed uninterrupted expression of their concerns to their doctor in their office visits. The second study indicated this same result, along with improvement in:

- Daily living skills
- Health status, as perceived by the patient
- Blood sugar control

Roter and Hall (Ref. #96) state that medical research indicates doctor-patient communication in general (involving patient education, counseling, behavioral medicine techniques, as well as verbal and nonverbal communication skills) is associated with:

- Improved postoperative recovery
- Decreased use of pain medication
- Shorter hospital stays

Communication Skills: Cognitive Processing Styles

As Herrmann states (Ref. #56), we may verbally state the same words, but put entirely different meaning or perspective on them due to our different cognitive processing preferences (Section #9). These differences in processing can be so great that mental language dialects are created. These are:

- The language of logic and reason: (facts - Upper Left)
- The language of structure and control: (form - Lower Left)
- The language of feelings and emotions: (feeling - Lower Right)
- The language of intuition and imagination: (future - Upper Right)

(See Section #9 for more information.)

How does this relate to communication? Generally, in the Herrmann Brain Dominance Instrument (Section #9), the quadrants diagonally opposed to each other symbolize the greatest gaps in communication.

For example, the national general profile of a psychiatrist is 2-2-2-1 (Ref. #56). That of a psychologist is 2-2-1-1 (Appendix B). Section #9 explains what the numbers mean and that each four number profile is to be read from upper left to upper right in a counter clockwise direction. A person who has a profile of 2-2-1-1 and whose dominant score is highest on the lower right probably would establish greater rapport with the psychologist than the psychiatrist, who has a "2" score for the Lower Right. A "2" indicates that the psychiatrist only recognizes the necessity for using that particular mode of processing but he/she doesn't prefer naturally to use it. This same person might also make greater progress with the psychologist if the need exists to unmask pent-up emotions, express them, and deal with their sources.

A surgeon has a national profile of 1-1-2-2. This person is not naturally going to be sensitive to the emotions, feelings, stress, and anxiety faced by a patient, particularly a patient who has a 2-2-1-1 profile. This type of patient is automatically going to perceive the surgeon as having terrible "bedside manners." A person with a profile of 1-2-2-3 is not going to be a high risk taker. In informed consent interviews, all the facts must be established and given with pros and cons of various options carefully explained. The specialist may have to give probabilities of success and give detailed reasons for his/her choice of treatment. A person with a profile of 2-2-1-1 is a high risk taker. A proper counseling technique to take with this person is a future orientation; for example: "Image yourself free of pain after this operation is performed. Imagine what you can accomplish with greater mobility. Imagine the feelings of relief you'll be feeling..."

For long-term patients, such as those with chronic pain, doctors should use a formalized assessment of the cognitive processing style(s) of the patient, such as use of the Herrmann Brain Dominance Instrument and/or the Myers-Briggs Personality Type Indicator. An awareness may help foster at least active listening skills and efforts to verbally address the patients' preferred mode(s) of processing information.

In short-term stays such as in acute care facilities, formalized assessment may be impractical. However, as stated in Section #9, there is a direct relationship between brain dominance occupational profile, and cognitive/learning preferences. Psychosocial data is given on patient charts. It doesn't take much time to ask a person what he/she does for a living, what his/her hobbies are, and/or what his/her favorite subjects were in school.

Given the proven reliability and validity of the assessed Herrmann Brain Dominance Instrument and the popularity of the Myers-Briggs, it makes sense to ask, as part of the history, if a patient has such results. If the healthcare provider is unfamiliar with these instruments and their importance to the communication process, the authors urge him/her to investigate them and consider their application - at least for him/herself.

Once Swartz was visiting a friend of his, a retired male stockbroker, in post-operative recovery immediately following back surgery. Coming into his private room, Swartz saw Paul in extreme nonverbal discomfort and agitation, throwing down fluff reading material. Thinking that it might be post-op pain, Swartz asked Paul if he should call for a nurse and then leave. Paul said no. But in a loud and frustrated voice, he uttered, "Why is all that confusion and chaos going on out there? I asked a nurse; she shrugged her shoulders and just left me [expletives deleted]!" Knowing that Paul had Lower Left and Lower Right cognitive preferences, Swartz first of all explained point by point that the chaos was fairly typical - it was "controlled [Lower Left] chaos" and that shift changes were starting. Paul then asked how the floor was organized [Lower Left needs]. Swartz explained, even volunteered to get an organization chart from Personnel/Human Resources so he could get a sense of how the positions at the nurses station related to other disciplines. This began to satisfy Paul and the stress and anxiety abated, without need for medication. Through explanation, Swartz was also recognizing Paul's need for social support and interpersonal expression of emotions [Lower Right]. The nurse failed to reach Paul's cognitive processing modes, contributing to his post-op stress level. Also, the nurse, by walking out of the room, failed to give some control [Lower Left] to the situation. Granted, Paul's request may have been atypical, but the nurse should have responded to the needs of the patient.

Communication Skills: Questioning

We previously mentioned that doctors, when questioning patients, frequently ask questions that solicit either a yes or no response. These are called *close-ended questions.*

An *open-ended question* (Section #8) is designed to solicit more information. It cannot be answered simply by yes or no. Asking "How do you feel?" and allowing for feedback and listening to what the patient is saying is certainly going to elicit more information than the close-ended question, "Do you feel good on the medication that I prescribed?" A close-ended question is likely to solicit a yes or no response especially if the patient is conditioned by society to:

- Accept a traditionally passive role in the presence of the authority represented by a doctor
- Fear being considered as a trouble maker by speaking up

Open-ended questions solicit self-disclosure. This means starting questions with...

- Who
- What
- When
- How
- Where
- Why

As Roter and Hall report (Ref. #96), such information gives the doctor data needed to provide the relevant information to the patient. By knowing what concerns the patient, the doctor can make the information he/she provides more relevant to the patient. Furthermore, this information is added to the data the doctor is accumulating for the medical diagnosis, the main task at hand. Such questions add to the trust-relationship and to patient satisfaction with his/her doctor.

Roter and Hall (Ref. #96) also report several studies that definitively indicate that communication skills are directly related to quality of care standards as set by medical professionals. The studies measured actual doctor performance against medical standards. Quality of care was judged high in those cases where the doctors utilized these communication skills:

- Giving information to the patients, including biomedical information
- Providing counseling
- Asking more open-ended questions and fewer close-ended questions

Task and process issues go hand-in-hand. *Task* is the *what*, the end result, that is to be performed. *Process* relates to the ways used to arrive at the end result. The medical diagnosis is the task; communication issues and patient education become part of the process.

Resources: Pertaining to the Herrmann Brain Dominance Instrument, see Section #31.

References (Sources cited in this section): 16, 17, 26, 38, 48, 51, 56, 60, 88, 93, 96, 103

References (Sources used as general reference works for this section): 6, 113

SELF-HEALTH SKILLS

Notes

#23: YOUR BELIEFS, YOUR HEALTH

Overview

Considering the extensive research on the impact of stress upon health (Section #17), Dr. Benson's research on the relaxation response (Section #18), and the clinical research from the field of psychoneuroimmunology (Section #14), it is evident that mind does play a major role in healing. But what role, if any, do attitudes and beliefs play in the healing process?

As Dr. Dossey states (Ref. #34), when confronted with illness and disease, we face one basic question: "How will I respond to this crisis?" Our belief system will help determine the answers.

The questions raised in Sections #14, #17 and #18 furnish the focus of this section.

The Faith Factor

Recall from Section #18 that prayer and meditation are two ways of evoking the relaxation response. This same section also listed the many physiological benefits derived from the relaxation response.

Dr. Herbert Benson, Director of the Mind/Body Medical Institute, Division of Behavioral Medicine, New England Deaconess Hospital (see Resources, Section #31), regards the use of prayer and meditation as very effective in attaining the relaxation response and its important physiological benefits. He called this the *faith factor* in his work, *Beyond the Relaxation Response* (Ref. #9). Dr. Benson, gives a detailed step-by-step exercise used in the Mind/Body Medical Institute to elicit the relaxation response through the faith factor. (See Ref. #48, Chapter 14, for this exercise.)

Optimism and Pessimism

The best research studies investigating optimism and pessimism link attitudes to behaviors (Ref. #48, Chapter 21). Optimistic individuals will tend to engage in wellness (health-promoting) behaviors such as:

- Proper nutrition
- Exercising

- Periodic medical examinations
- Being actively involved with their doctors in the treatment process when confronted with disease

Pessimistic people will tend to be socially isolated. This isolation becomes a risk factor (Section #24). Furthermore they tend to seek out similar people when they do seek support. Thus, by peer pressure, surrounded and reinforced by negative people, these individuals have an even harder time of changing their negative attitudes. Recall from Section #17 that one of the emotional impacts of chronic stress is feeling helpless and/or hopeless. This feeling develops when one perceives that the stressor(s) he/she is faced with is/are stronger than the resources available to cope with the problem. Negative people help feed negative perceptions. Hence, a self-fulfilling prophecy emerges and assumes a life of its own.

Hardiness, Helplessness, Hope and Blame

The concept of hardiness to stress is related to an optimistic attitude. Recall from Section #18 that the degree of hardiness to stressors is dependent upon three key components:

- Commitment to values
- Control over events
- Challenge

An optimistic attitude fosters belief in resources available to cope with or solve a problem. *Dispositional optimism* is defined as the degree to which an individual expects more positive events to happen rather than negative events (Ref. #48, Chapter 21). Is there a relationship to physical health? Researchers have found that when studying patients' recovery rates following coronary artery bypass surgery, those with a predisposition toward optimistic attitudes were more likely to have:

- Returned to work
- Resumed past social, sexual and recreational activities as compared to those patients holding more negative attitudes (Ref. #48, Chapter 21)

Guilt and shame produce low self esteem. The lack of self-esteem lays the foundation for psychological helplessness: The conscious knowledge that I, having no control over a situation, will initially fear the situation. This initial fear leads to depression.

Also involved in helplessness is the loss of hope. Researchers identify two components of hopefulness (Ref. #48, Chapter 21):

- Having the ability to create plans to meet goals
- Having the self-determination to meet goals

Hope fosters health, as studies have shown. Thus it may be important for healthcare providers to maintain an illusion to clients - at least initially - until their clients can accept this attitude:

Acceptance of a disease
is not *abnegation* to the disease.

An example: The facts say I have cancer. I accept it. However this does not mean that I necessarily have to die from it. I could be one of the survivors. If physical long-term cure is not possible, how can I enhance the quality of my remaining years? In what other areas of my life can I experience healing?

Low self-esteem pervades blame, consciously and/or subconsciously (See "Blame", Table 23.1, in this chapter).

If we are lame, we need a crutch upon which to be lame. The crutch can be our internal sense of guilt and shame (real or neurotic); others in our society and our environment (such as our parents); fate; chance; Satan; or even God.

Borysenko (Ref. #13) cites psychological studies that show how low self-esteem impacts religious beliefs (see below). Guilt-ridden pessimistic people (low self-esteem) described God as punitive and punishing. People with high self-esteem (self love, self trust) described God as a God of Love. Our perception of God is dependent upon our psychological state.

People having a high sense of self-esteem really do have an ego. In Swartz's counseling experience, the clients who made progress in alleviating their self-administered guilt and shame were the ones who made progress in self-growth, in developing a sense of ego, and in developing self-acceptance. The people we call egocentric are more often than not overcompensating for a lack of ego. These are the people whistling while walking past the graveyard. Individuals who lack a secure sense of self should work to develop an ego. Self-centeredness, for Swartz, is ego growth leading to self-acceptance, self-pride, and humility.

We can and perhaps should, at times, blame ourselves for real guilt and shame. But there comes a time when what is needed is to throw away the crutch. (See "Lesson", Table 23.1.) When we have learned our lesson, we have less on our chest and shoulders as burdens.

Self-centeredness (the development of self-esteem through ego growth) leads to development of hardiness and hope. Egocentrism (the lack of self-esteem due to the lack of ego) perpetuates blame and fosters helplessness. In this psychological dysfunctional state, we have even raised God from the dead. From "God is dead" a few decades ago, we have now created "God as co-dependent".

Hostility

In the 1960s, cardiologists Meyer Friedman and Ray Rosenman investigated possible connections of mind and coronary heart disease (CHD). They found a cluster of behavioral characteristics common to most patients with CHD. These characteristics were combined and coined "Type A" behavior (Ref. #43). This behavior involves these characteristics:

- Hyperaggressiveness
- A sense of insecurity
- Constant time urgency
- Free-floating hostility (permanent internal anger or rage)

Most well-designed 1970s and 1980s research studies still support the connection of hostility to CHD, though several researchers would agree that better ways are needed to identify and measure hostility (Ref. #48, Chapter 4). Regardless of how it is measured, pent-up hostility seems to increase the amount of stress hormones circulating in the blood stream. One of the stress hormones, adrenaline, raises blood pressure, contributes to accelerated blood clotting, and speeds the growth of *plaque*: deposits within the artery walls that build up over time. Plaque contributes to artherosclerosis, or hardening of the arteries. Adrenaline sets off the movement of stored body fat, containing nutrients that the body needs in a time of crisis, into the bloodstream. This raises the levels of blood cholesterol that accumulate as plaque.

The Importance of Spiritual Beliefs

Spiritual beliefs are the intrinsic beliefs an individual holds, regardless of his/her religion. By contrast, *religion* is an organized set of tenets.

To determine your own spiritual beliefs, ask yourself these important questions:

- Whose beliefs are they?
- Are they really mine or are they hand-me-downs from my past upbringing?
- What do I really believe?

Medical studies have been conducted on spiritual beliefs and their impact upon physical and psychological health. For example, religious beliefs have been found to be central for many people coping with cancer. Such beliefs evolve around finding meaning in their lives (Ref. #48, Chapter 5). Dr. Dossey (Ref. #35) cites a study investigating the impact of prayer upon surgical patients with coronary heart disease. The findings were that those patients being prayed for (without the staff or the patients knowing what was included in the experimental treatment [prayer group]) differed from those not being prayed for in several respects. The patients being prayed for:

- Had five times less need for antibiotics
- Were three times less likely to develop pulmonary edema (lungs filling with fluids)
- Had no need for endotracheal intubation (insertion of an artificial airway)

As Dr. Dossey states, we need to rediscover the soul and integrate it into modern medicine

Regardless of their direct effect on physical health, the authors feel that spiritual beliefs are critical for wellness programming and healing. Spiritual beliefs:

- Provide meaningfulness to our lives
- Represent one of the four levels of health
- Are a foundation for lower right cognitive processors (Sec. #9)
- Impact both guilt and shame

Meaning. Recall from above and Section #18 that one of the key components of stress management is hardiness. One of the primary ingredients of hardiness is commitment to values. Values are intrinsic motivators. In this materialistic, seemingly amoral society, values, and beliefs are the few "non-things" we can put inside us. We cannot put computers, cars, and other physical space items within us. What we do put inside are their values - what they represent to us. Beliefs help provide meaning to a life increasingly devoid of meaning.

Gartner, et al, found in a meta-analysis of several research studies that religious beliefs and spiritual beliefs are positively correlated (Ref. #94). People having strong religious beliefs:

- Have lower suicide rates
- Have lower drug use
- May have lower rate of delinquency (though the studies' results are mixed on this factor)
- Have generally happier marriages and lower divorce rates
- Have better mental illness recovery
- Express a sense of general well-being and satisfaction with life

Spiritual health. Spiritual beliefs represent a level of health. Within the full spectrum of healing as a movement towards wholeness, spiritual health represents inner control, removed from physical disability. The inner **I** is the eternal witness that is removed from the physical and psychological chaos going on within me. Recall that control is also a key component of hardiness. The more control I have, the more resources I can bring into a situation.

Within spiritual health, "nonlocal" mind has a chance of encountering "nonlocal" God. Physical things have a time-space orientation. Mind transcends both time and space. Within all major religions, one of the attributes of God is transcendence of time and space (Appendix D). In the silence of prayer and/or meditiation, I can meet God and arrive at an understanding that I am more than the confines of my physical body. The sounds of silence can be deafening.

What freedom! What liberation! I exist apart from the body. Yes, I witness the physical body as I am physically attached to it. Yet I am detached from it! This is balance: attached, yet detached. ("Balance", Table 23.1.)

A belief in the literal interpretation of these words, "I have cancer" leads to emphasis upon the existence of physical health only. A belief in wellness programming and the four levels of health leads to this statement: "The body has cancer." Which of these statements is closer to your beliefs? Which of these statements leads to hope and healing?

Cognitive processing: Section #9 explained that one of the key descriptors for a lower right processor is spiritual. This style of processing is one of four major ways of consciously processing information. For this style of thinker and learner, the incorporation of spirituality within health is important .

Impacting upon guilt and shame. In Section #5 the interrelationship of levels of health with one another was explained. The spiritual level also impacts the emotional level. This section describes how guilt and shame produce low self-esteem, a description of a God who needs to punish for committed sins.

In Swartz' counseling experience, the co-therapists who make progress are those who first identify their spiritual beliefs. Realization of a loving God occurs first on the part of the co-therapist. Then and only then is permission given internally to grow, after the co-therapist's ego accepts this self-given permission. Given this permission, with religious barriers that were contributing to guilt and shame having been removed, then and only then can the emotional issues be addressed. This has been a fascinating, consistent pattern to observe and it has tremendous implications in both psychoanalytical and psychological counseling. In allopathic medicine, not enough attention has been paid to the interrelationship of spiritual beliefs, guilt and shame. In Asian religions and psychologies, "Self is teacher, ego is pupil".

Table 23.1

LANGUAGE LESSON WORDS

(Words in our language carry lessons inherent in them: - "Lesson words")

Balance: B(e) al(l) an(d) ce(see)
Believe: "Be" and "live"
Blame: B(e) lame
Ignorance: Ignore an(d) ce(see)
Lesson: Less on
Responsibility: Respond ability
Sin: See in

The Importance of Quality

This section has given reasons why spiritual beliefs are important to healing and wellness. But does the quality of these beliefs matter? Clearly explained in this section, the quality of emotional beliefs impact both physical and spiritual levels of health. From the psychological studies referred to, people with high self-esteem relate to a God of love, those with low self-esteem relate to, or even need, a punishing God. How do spiritual beliefs affect health? Can a God of love reinforce a sense of self-esteem? Can a God of wrath reinforce a sense of low self-esteem? For the authors, Dossey (Refs. #34 and #35), Borysenko (Ref. #13), et al, the answer to these last two questions is yes.

Not only is it important to have spiritual beliefs, it is equally important for the co-therapist to determine for his/herself the quality of his/her beliefs and investigate the emotions intertwined with those beliefs.

There are two basic emotions: love and fear. Each of these is interrelated, as we have seen, with spiritual beliefs. Each has produced almost two different theologies based upon two different needs: a God of love and a God of wrath.

Fear-Based Spiritual Beliefs

The crux of fear-based spiritual beliefs is a God of wrath: "God is punishing me for my sins. I am even unworthy of God's love. I deserve to be damned for eternity."

The foundation for this premise is a time-oriented God. This chronological time orientation has as its postulates:

- God as creator
- Original sin
- A quid pro quo co-dependency
- The future is heaven, hell, or some sense of purgatory

God as creator. God created the universe.

Original sin. There was a fall from grace. Humanity sinned. All members of the human race are born into sin.

Quid pro quo co-dependency. In this concept, God definitely acts in time. "God punishes me for my sins when I am bad. I will be rewarded if I am good" (following the laws, observing the sacraments, commandments, etc.). God's actions depend upon, are co-dependent with, the acts and actions of the individual. This leads to a time-oriented future in heaven or hell, or some sense of purgatory. (For further elaboration, see Appendix E.)

Consequences of Fear-Based Spiritual Beliefs

As Borysenko states (Ref. #13), it is easier to place blame on a person or thing than to accept the helplessness of a situation. At least with blame, a person or thing is in control. And, as atheists and agnostics might say, humanity needs to feel in control; that is why we invented God.

But what of the concept of change? In this framework of beliefs, change becomes excruciatingly difficult. The therapist can create the environment allowing for the possibility of self-motivation but ultimately the responsibility for change resides in the co-therapist. At best, the co-therapist will perhaps ask for relief of symptoms when they get bad enough but not for cure or healing of the cause(s) creating the symptoms. God created original sin. Rather than tenets, such statements and phrases become permanent concrete shackles holding the person.

God punishes. Therefore, I fear him/her, Jehovah, Yahweh, Supreme Being, etc. I will therefore carry out to the letter the literal interpretation of the commandment/law/sacrament. I will not question. I will rely solely upon others to interpret and tell me what to do. The only interrelationship here between Creator and created is that of fear. Growth cannot be sustained in a state of fear. Furthermore, a state of fear leads to a state of isolation, abandonment, a fear of rejection and, ultimately, aloneness. The universe is not a friendly place to live.

Two chief emotions arise from fear. One is hate. The other is aloneness. Consider our society's emphasis upon materialism, being socially acceptable, and doing anything to escape being alone, including being immersed in, or surrounded by, technology.

Love-Based Spiritual Beliefs

The crux of love-based spiritual beliefs is a God of love and charity. The external manifestation is growth on the part of the individual.

Appendices D and E provide information on spiritual beliefs. We, the authors, ask the reader to compare his/her own beliefs to those listed.

The tenets of love-based beliefs reside in "the perennial philosophy", a term coined by the philosopher Leibnitz. Appendix D, "Principles of the Perennial Philosophy," contains a summary of the commonalities found in all major religions, as they are explained in two classic works (Refs. #58 and #101). The perennial principles listed in Appendix D are the core for spiritual beliefs based on a God of love (Refs. #42 and #106). By contrast, Appendix E, "Implications of a Time-Oriented God for Health and Healing," explains the core of fear-based spiritual beliefs that were

previously described in this section.
Two types of time exist: kairological and chronological. *Kairological* is defined as "a time when conditions are right for the accomplishment of a crucial action: the opportune and decisive moment." (Webster's 3rd New International Dictionary [G&C Merriam Company, Springfield, MA] 1981, p. 1230.)

A God of love and the implications of love-based spiritual beliefs and healing operate in kairological timelessness. By contrast, fear-based spiritual beliefs interact with a God based in chronological time. Appendix E lists the health consequences of belief in a God based on chronological time.

In love-based spiritual beliefs, God is both within and without, manifesting in time while remaining timeless. A timeless God never stops creating. Thus change is not only possible, it is occurring. My condition in life is not permanent and change can occur if I can overcome my fear associated with change. The "perennial philosophy" gives rise to spiritual optimism, not pessimism. Individuals feel more a part of God, not apart from God.

Love-based spiritual beliefs lead to growth and give rise to another interpretation of "original sin". ("Sin and ignorance", Table 23.1.) The original sin is the failure to see into myself and examine my own actions, thoughts, and emotions. By ignoring the internal, I am bound to keep repeating the same mistakes over and over. I will see the consequences of each situation but will not see the overall pattern and the causes. Only when I become aware and break the pattern will I be able to change. It is interesting that the root meaning of the word *sin* originally meant missing the mark, separation (Refs. #101 and #106).

How does love-based healing operate in kairological timelessness? Recall the phrase "Only when I become aware and break the pattern..." One symbolic meaning of the Christian cross is that the horizontal bar of the cross represents chronological time and the vertical represents timeless, potential kairological time. Consider that the moment of my insight, my seeing in, my awareness of my acts, emotions, and thoughts and how they can be contributing to my pattern occurs when the two halves of the cross "cross." This is the moment of crucifixion, my moment of health. Do I crucify myself by mortifying (cutting off; pruning) my ego or do I ignore this insight and keep on repeating the same behaviors or patterns?

A God of love does not mean an absence of universal structure. This initial "seeing in" is essential for repentance. Forgiveness of myself follows. These steps must occur before I can take responsibility for myself. Instead of blaming others, I must understand how my own actions have contributed to my present situation and take responsibility for them.

Love-based beliefs also have an answer to this often-asked question: "If God is love and I am good, why do bad things happen to good people?" This question originates from duality ("Wellness," Sec. #18) and the need for control in our lives.

A major precept of the perennial philosophy is that if good things exist, bad things must also exist. If happiness exists, pain and suffering must exist. To experience health and to understand it, individuals have to experience an unhealthy (lack of health) disease and illness. This provides a balanced comparison. When we have health we should appreciate it. This is what Eastern religions mean when they say "live in the present." To put this another way:

Continuum subsumes *duality*: either/or

We need to appreciate what we have, for it will change. We need to appreciate life, for death is a part of life. We need to appreciate pleasures and happiness, for pain and suffering are a part of happiness. The Western Judeo-Christian world is so dualistic, time-oriented and materialistic that life is based on gratifying future-oriented desires. Often only at death do we realize that we missed life. That is one reason death is so fearful to us.

Although many things are beyond our control, we need to take responsibility for changing the things we can control. The relationship between developing lung cancer and smoking three packs of cigarettes a day for 35 years is obvious. Also obvious is the relationship between sexual promiscuity and developing HIV and AIDS. The person who builds a house on a diversified flood plain must face the likely consequences of flooding.

Consequences of Love-Based Spiritual Beliefs

Love-based spiritual health puts you in the frame of mind where healing can occur. The following result:

- Your emotions are more in balance. The mood swings are not as low or as high. You are on a more even keel
- With this balance, you become more detached from your environment and its stressors. Your emotional energy is better utilized, rather than wasting your energy, being invested in, consumed by your stressors
- By retaining more control, you develop hardiness to stress

(It's a fascinating process; by giving up control, you gain more control.)
- You do develop self-discipline
- You give meaning to your existence

Conclusion

In a time of health crisis, your beliefs - psychological and spiritual - will determine how you respond to that crisis. Beliefs based upon psychological and spiritual pessimism will help contribute to your sense of isolation, your sense of hopelessness and helplessness, and to the illness: the stress accompanying the physiological disease. Beliefs based upon psychological and spiritual optimism will give you resources to cope with both your physical disease and your stressors. It is your health and, given free will, your choice.

We, the authors, only urge that you not wait until a time of crisis to sort out your beliefs. Recall above that only beliefs and values can be put inside you - not your material possessions. This is like putting money into a bank, or building up a stock portfolio. The financial resources are there when needed. Invest in yourself, open up a beliefs account, so you can draw upon them when needed. Finally, see "Believe", Table 23.1.

References: 9, 13, 34, 35, 42, 43, 48, 58, 94, 101, 106

#24: SOCIAL SUPPORT

Introduction: a Nation of Isolation - Healthcare as Aloneness

Beliefs and values are intrinsic to the individual. As seen in Section #23, beliefs (including spiritual) and emotions impact both physical cure and healing. These internal forces have a great effect on health.

Much research exists to demonstrate that external forces, such as social support, directly impact physical cure and healing. Social support has been defined in terms of quality, not quantity: how well people meet your needs (Ref. #48, Chapter 20).

In spite of this alleged age of communication, we tend to be an increasingly isolated society. The violence in our society forces us to be at home with our doors locked. Technology via the information highway brings our entertainment to us but creates an environment conducive to non-communication; it is simply easier to "veg out" and "watch the tube". The telephone, the word processor, the fax, the computer, and electronic mail communicate the words but not the nonverbal language that gives hidden meaning to those words. Dysfunctional families exhibiting abuse and violence within the home remind us that even locked doors are not enough.

We are a nation of technological nomads. We increasingly travel farther and farther to our jobs in daily commutes. Many individuals reject car pooling because the car with one driver is one of the last bastions of feeling in control and being allowed to be alone. We change jobs constantly in pursuit of our careers and the faded American Dream. Our suburban communities are stylized "bedroom communities." Highways, corporate office buildings, malls and satellite cities at exit ramps have replaced suburbs, which have replaced neighborhoods.

A sense of community is increasingly hard to find, much less maintain. Our history and our culture, paying homage to the myth of the rugged individual, reinforces this increased sense of isolation. Men are still taught not to display emotions. In our culture, we are not taught how to communicate in relationships - any relationship. A marriage license does not require hours spent in counseling and communication training; no such prerequisites for obtaining a license exist. A divorce decree represents the lack of such requirements. The sounds of silence are deafening.

In our culture, mass media advertising programs us into what to do, not how to think. Communication requires empathetic and active listening skills as well as critical thinking skills. Such communication skills are not valued in a society that worships the god of consumption served by the archangel technology. Reasoning is difficult in the "Nine Second Sound Byte Age" with the short attention span held by the mass audience.

Medical schools reinforce this by not training their students in communication skills. A student may not even see a live patient until his/her third year (Ref. #60).

Third party payers reimburse for the diagnosis but not for time spent in counseling or in communicating with the patient in the process of determining a diagnosis. Thus third party payers reinforce isolation.

Illness and disease reinforce isolation. The sick draw away from the healthy. The healthy, lacking basic communication skills to begin with and uncomfortable with physical proximity to the sick, perhaps fearing for their own mortality, draw back from the sick. Visiting hours bring tremendous amounts of stress, with both the patient and the family visitor unable to communicate effectively in this healthcare setting.

Most hospital waiting rooms reinforce isolation. Waiting room environments are cold and bleak, with old and worn copies of magazines. In coldness and in isolation, drawn inward by their own fears, the family members of the patients gather and "wait it out". Cold, stark silence and fear felt by one communicates with the silence of another. The sounds of silence are indeed deafening.

But there is hope. When social support is fostered, healing takes place.

Clinical Research

Dr. David Spiegel of Stanford University's School of Medicine did landmark research, begun in 1976, regarding the impact of social support on women with breast cancer (Ref. #48, Chapter 20). His research team organized the women into randomly selected support groups (the experimental group) and a group receiving then prescribed medical treatment (the control group). They found that the quality of life of the experimental group significantly improved over the control group. The experimental group also received medical treatment, including pain management via self-hypnosis; the control group did not receive such organized social support. The women in experimental social support groups used the groups as a structured vehicle to vent their emotions.

Regarding quality of life, the researchers specifically found that the women in the experimental groups:

- Collectively addressed ways to improve communication with their doctors (Section #8)
- Left unproductive relationships
- Became more emotionally stable and less depressed as compared to those in the control groups, who displayed increasingly disturbed moods
- Reported 50 percent less pain than the control group
- Became friends with one another, helping each other deal with their fears and deal with difficult family members
- Helped each other to die

Regarding longevity, the researchers were surprised to find that those in the experimental group lived an average of 18 months longer than those in the control group. In the first four years from the initiation of this study, none of the control group was alive; one third of the experimental group were. As of 1991, two of the women in the experimental group were still living. Dr. Spiegel states that he was surprised at the findings. He was not looking for such life extension and did not believe it would happen (Ref. #48, Chapter 20).

Other large-scale studies have produced similar results: an increase in both quality and quantity of life. These studies have not only involved different types of cancer patients but also those experiencing coronary heart disease (CHD). For example, in one study, perceived inferior social support by married men with CHD increased the chance of hospital readmission (Ref. #25).

Ornstein and Sobel (Ref. #81) report studies indicating that interventions to reinforce and strengthen social support improve medical treatment compliance and mortality. One study found a 57 percent decline in the experimental group's death rate compared to that of the control group.

One of the mega-analysis research studies referred to in Section #2 found that patient education reduces healthcare cost by reducing length of hospital stay by a mean average of 1.25 days (Ref. #33). Social support was one of the behavioral treatments common to all studies included in the mega-analysis.

It is not simply persons with acute health problems who have been studied. Studies involving thousands of men and women have found that those who are divorced have more health problems than those who are widowed, married, or single. However, being married is not the cure for all problems. Six national studies have found that individuals who are unhappy in their marriages have poorer health than those who report being contented in their marriages (Ref. #48, Chapter 20).

Married men live longer and have less physical disease than men who are divorced, widowed, or single. They also report being emotionally happier. Divorced and widowed men tend to remarry quickly (Ref. #81).

Married women have higher rates of mental illness and depression than married men. Married men react more strongly to the loss (via death) of their wives than women do to the loss of their husbands. Widowers experience three times the death rate of widows (Ref. #81). Why? Men are trained in this culture to have these three characteristic traits associated with masculinity (Ref. #25):

- Lack of empathy
- Lack of emotional expression
- Increased social isolation

The Ned Herrmann Group's data base (as of 1993) of approximately 75,000 individual Brain Dominance Instrument profiles (Section #9 and Reference #56) indicates distinct communication differences between males and females. According to this data base, Herrmann's research indicates that women generally have a natural tendency to use the lower right quadrant in cognitive processing as compared to men. Recall from Section #9 that the lower right quadrant relates to communication and expression of feelings. This corresponds to, and positively correlates with, several popular books of recent years concerning communication differences between the sexes.

Women are much more likely to develop support networks and lifelong friends than men. Hence, women's bonded friendships and support networks help them in time of loss. For men, generally, their closest friend and confidant is their spouse. Also, for men, their friendships are prone to be situational and time-oriented: built around hobbies, work, sports, school, etc. (Ref. #81). When the interest is past, the work changes, or the schooling is over, males tend to move on, leaving friendship with other males.

Healing and Pets

Incidentally, quality social support does not come only from people. Dr. Spiegel

(Ref. #48, Chapter 20) cites several medical studies indicating that pet ownership facilitates healing, especially for those owners who love their pets and do not simply possess them. These studies found the following:

- Comparing people discharged from a coronary care unit, pet owners survived longer than those not having pets
- As a predictor of survival, pet ownership was stronger than having a spouse or family social support
- A study of elderly pet owners indicated that pet owners saw a physician fewer times in a year than elderly patients having no pets

Perhaps other factors are at play here. Pet ownership, especially where the owner truly loves the pet, is a manifestation of love-based spiritual beliefs (Sec. #24). However, certainly a loved pet is a resource giving meaning to the owner's existence. Recall that commitment is one of the major components in developing hardiness to stress (Ref. #81).

Why Does Social Support "Work"?

The differences between the sexes offer consequences in terms of the organization and structure of social support groups. Men need help in increasing their communication skills and in learning to express emotions before tackling the specific emotions and problems related to a disease within the parameters of a social support group. Women bond more quickly than men. Women and the concept of social support are a more natural fit. Social support groups composed entirely of women are more effective. Other reasons why social support is effective, in terms of obtaining the results reported under "Clinical research" above, are outlined as follows.

Social support influences behavior, which impacts physical health. People who know loved ones care about them, are more likely to reduce bad health habits such as drug use, unsafe sex, excessive drinking, and inadequate nutrition.

People who have good interpersonal skills and are communication-oriented also have better rapport and communication with healthcare professionals. Recall from Section #8 that doctors and their staffs who perceive that the patients are communicating with them will tend to reinforce this behavior by giving this type of patient more information.

People who communicate with each other and help each other also simultaneously help reduce their own stress level. This reduces the amount of stress hormones in the bloodstream (Section #17) and this aids their immune system. In addition, remember that stress differs from individual to individual due to the concept of hardiness each individual has developed. Recall that three major components to hardiness are (Section #18):

- Control
- Challenge
- Commitment

The greater the resources, the greater the sense of control. People are resources. These resources include such diverse groups as: patients in a support group, the staff involved in running the support group, the caregiver(s), friends, etc.

In a support group, the client is taught to take responsibility for his/her *healing*, not necessarily physical cure. Recall the four levels of health (Section #5). If physical cure comes about, terrific. There are options, even if one has a terminal disease. Finally, in a support group, the co-therapists share with and support one another. In this way, they provide meaning in their lives because they are committed to one another. A sense of isolation, leading to hopelessness and helplessness, is replaced by a sense of community.

Patient Education as Social Support

Dr. Spiegel (Ref. #48, Chapter 20) identifies four major types of social support groups:

- Social support
- Emotional ventilation
- Cognitive restructuring
- Education

His research study (see above, in "Clinical research") utilized the first two approaches. Cognitive restructuring involves helping the client first become aware of his/her perception of a situation and the assumptions, other beliefs and values underlying that perception. This is helping the client change his/her perception (a paradigm shift). Given this new awareness, then the therapy helps the client develop appropriate behavioral responses to the situation as the client now perceives it.

The Learning Center of the University of Minnesota Hospital and Clinic (Table 10.1, Section #10) studied the impact of patient education upon preparing patients in home self-care. Their findings were as follows (Ref. #47):

- The number of learning outcomes achieved were higher for those patients trained at the Learning Center (in the proper use of right atrial catheters) than for those patients not attending formalized training at the Center

- The number of hospital readmissions related to catheter complications and/or catheter reinsertions were lower for those attending formalized training at the Learning Center than for those not attending such formalized training

Both Spiegel and Goldstein place value on patient education as a social support. Patient education conducted as formalized training involving groups of patients having common objectives constitutes a social support group. One of the reasons for the results listed in Section #2 is that patient education is social support, whether conducted one-on-one or in formalized groups. Also, as previously noted, research has found social support to be effective in healing.

Patient education thus simultaneously serves two major functions:

- It offers training and education to clients (while giving them the opportunity to be co-therapists in the sense of assuming greater responsibility for self-care in disease and treatment)
- It facilitates social support while assisting in physical cure and healing

By performing these two functions, the field of patient education serves as a cost containment strategy (Section #2).

Consequences for Patient Education

Both the Spiegel research cited above and the University of Minnesota Hospital and Clinic Learning Center have documented the value of patient education as a support group versus formalized training. If the Learning Center's results (Refs. 46 and #47) are replicated consistently, it would be wise to cluster patients with common objectives into formalized training programs.

Consumer Tips: Elements of Positive Support Groups

The following tips are intended for the lay person seeking social support on his/her own and for the healthcare professional interested in starting support groups, including patient education, or referring clientele to support groups.

1. Seek out support. A person confronted with major disease and illness has two basic choices: (1) isolation, that can lead to hopelessness and helplessness; (2) active participation in wellness programming (Section #18) that can assist in healing, if not physical cure. The latter involves social support. Because our

society and culture, and illness and disease itself, naturally tend to isolate us, we have to guard against, even fight, isolation tendencies.

2. Select the support group that will be most helpful to you. Support groups whose emphasis is social support and emotional ventilation are not for you, if:

- You are not trained in self-disclosure
- You dislike sharing your feelings (such as being a very left brain oriented cognitive processor - Section #9)
- You are not interested in others

In selecting a group, ask the following questions:

- Are these current feelings really me or due to the disease and illness I am experiencing?
- Could I benefit more from patient education groups?
- Am I denying the existence of a disease or illness that I don't wish to hear about?
- Am I afraid of hearing about consequences of my disease or illness?

3. Prior to attending your first meeting, work out the answers to these questions: What am I willing to divulge at this point? What are the things I do not wish to share? What are my ground rules going in?

4. Some things to look for when you attend a meeting are these:

- Who is in charge? Is the group facilitated by trained group facilitators? Do they involve patients (co-therapists) having what I've experienced? Do they involve professional staff? Have they had prior experience in working with support groups?
- Are any members of the group belittled, put down in any way for what they say or don't say? Is this encouraged by the facilitator? If so, don't come back. Seek out another group
- Is the focus of the group healing or strictly physical cure? (Section #5)
- Is there any blaming the victim gamesmanship permitted? (Section #7) If so, don't come back
- Is the group *so* positive in its orientation or attitude (i.e., you will be cured physically) that it becomes Pollyanna? Acceptance of a disease is not abnegation to it. Acceptance of outcomes can be healing. If the group is dealing in Pollyanna, does/do the facilitator(s) encourage it and allow it to continue?
- What resources, if any, are provided the members between meetings? If you have a major problem and feel you need help, will you have anyone to

call? When?
- Do the facilitators practice what they preach? This may not be apparent by the end of your first meeting

5. Explore the following resources:
    - Your hospital's patient education coordinator
    - Your doctor
    - Voluntary organizations such as the American Heart Association and American Cancer Society

Additional resources are listed in Section #31 of this book.

Finally, for those healthcare professionals involved in patient education, the authors advocate at least, if not formal orientation sessions, development and distribution of printed information for the basic family and the primary caregivers on how to give proper social support. Such tips range from the need to discuss what you are feeling through the importance of sharing and not holding back secrets. Such information should also contain tips for the family members on giving information to people who call and why it is important to conserve caregivers' energy and resources.

References: 25, 33, 47, 48, 56, 60, 81

#25: THE HOME HEALING ENVIRONMENT

Overview

If responsibility for healing is not taken in the hospital, it must surely be taken at home. Furthermore, the need for home healthcare is increasing. Patients are being discharged from the hospital "sicker and quicker". This trend will continue. Following hospital discharge, the work of recuperation is just beginning; but now it is without the 24-hour technical support services received at the hospital. The co-therapist and the caregiver have three major areas of responsibility during the recuperation period following discharge:

1. Establishing and maintaining a physical environment conducive to healing
2. Increasing the quality of social support
3. Implementing stress management and wellness

1. Establishing and maintaining a physical environment conducive to healing. The physical environment includes all of the following factors:

- Lighting
- Natural environment
- Music and sound
- Organization and structure
- Color

These factors, particularly the first three, are conducive to healing as well as learning. They help create the relaxation response (Section #18) and for learning, a state of being relaxed, yet alert (Ref. #103). Also refer to the discussion of music and sound in Section #21.

Lighting. Early in the 1980s, a Harris poll indicated that out of all office workers surveyed, 85 percent identified lighting as the number one factor in on-the-job comfort (Ref. #72). Lighting should be comfortable and adequate, avoiding problems associated with glare. Lighting appropriate for a 25-year-old may have too much glare for a person aged 45 and above (Ref. #72).

As much as possible, lighting should be natural, with your physical location in close proximity to a window. Studies have found that natural lighting in the work place actually helps people feel better (Ref. #72). What is true for the office is true for both the hospital and home healing environment.

Unfortunately, hospital rooms with views may be the exception and not the rule. Ornstein and Sobel (Ref. #82) reported that one environmental study of hospitals found this last statement to be true. They also cited a study contrasting patients who experienced a similar surgery (gall bladder). In this study, patients having a window overlooking nature compared to those with a window facing a brick wall:

- Spent almost one less day in the hospital post surgery
- Needed less pain medication
- Experienced fewer postoperative problems with nausea and headache

If natural lighting is impossible, the next best alternative is full spectrum lighting. This type of fluorescent bulb simulates natural light, providing the ultraviolet and visible parts of the light spectrum (Ref. #3) similar to the full spectrum of sunlight. Some studies suggest that such lighting may improve visual acuity and contribute to office productivity by making work less fatiguing (Refs. #73 and #108). (A negative side effect may be exposure to ultraviolet light, associated with skin cancer.)

Avoid direct overhead fluorescent lighting whenever possible. Fluorescent lighting flickers at approximately 120 times every second, faster than the eye can see. Recent research with Video Display Terminal (VDT) workers indicates that this type of lighting causes fatigue (Ref. #108). Studies have also found other health impairments associated with direct fluorescent lighting. They include (Refs. #3 and #72):

- Muscle soreness
- Headache
- Eye strain

Most environmental psychologists and lighting experts recommend ambient indirect lighting, another form of fluorescent lighting. Indirect lighting, caused by light fixtures bouncing light off the ceiling, appears to help reduce contrast ratios on architectural surfaces. The existence of a high *contrast ratio* (the difference in brightness between an object and its background) can produce the same physiological symptoms as fluorescent lighting (Refs. #3, #72, and #108).

Natural environment. Over the last eight years, in conducting relaxation training associated with accelerated learning, patient education, and stress management, Swartz has asked participants to write down the place where ultimate relaxation is found. This question is posed before any discussion or practice of relaxation training. He has found that 90 percent of any audience, no matter what the age, race, or part of the country, will list an out-of-doors scene. If a place is indoors, water is usually associated with it.

It is a given fact that nature helps us relax. The innate intelligence of the body knows where it needs to be to be relaxed. Yet with our urban development, we are getting farther and farther away from nature. Such development is isolating us even from our own body's need to have a place, a sanctuary, where our bodies can truly relax. Through senseless, unplanned urban sprawl, with our "if it sways in a breeze, pave it" mentality, we are slowly poisoning ourselves with additional artificial environmental stressors: from music (and what passes to be music) and noise (Section #21) through neon technology and concrete. We who call ourselves sensual have become "asensual". We who revere artificial intelligence are artificial, becoming that which we revere. It seems that the only thing we consistently strive for is natural regularity. We don't walk in mown grass; we smoke grass. Our drug culture has given a new connotation to the term "high school".

How artificial are we? Try turning off the television set for two weeks and begin to interact with your family. It is difficult.

Can an artificial environment be instrumental in the amoral violence exhibited more and more by today's young?

Consider this: The child is programmed with switches and buttons. He/she is progressively exposed, without structure or discipline, to violence and noise (Section #21) in television and movies through music videos and video games. Furthermore, all these stimuli are fast paced. This promotes and programs into the youngster quick and reactive stimulus-response actions. He/she is programmed to react spontaneously through physical manipulation of his/her environment.

Don't like something? Hit the remote switches. Like something? Replay it. Nothing dies. It is simply turned off and on through switches and buttons. This environment is artificial. Only the senses of seeing, hearing, and touching on a conscious level are involved. The other person in his/her environment is an object existing solely for his/her manipulation and control.

Consider this question: How many children and adolescents who pull the trigger on someone who instantly displeases them really feel they don't kill anyone but simply turn it off?

Research studies have conclusively shown that a young child cannot distinguish movies, television, etc., from reality.

Furthermore, such media directly contribute to violence. Swartz feels that our technological culture and media, plus its emphasis on violence combined with totally inappropriate music, inhibits both the development of left brain thinking and critical thinking skills. For example, chronological time (a cognitive function of the left hemisphere [Sections #9 and #7 of Ref. #103]) - time to think - is needed while contemplating future consequences of one's actions. Media (utilizing imagery) and its accompanying music help produce spontaneous reactions - physically and emotionally. Imagery and timelessness are functions of the right brain hemisphere (Sections #9 and #7 of Ref. #103). Music impacts the right hemisphere, thus reinforcing the right hemisphere's functions involving imagery and timelessness.

If you, the reader, do not believe this is true, then ask yourself these questions: What type(s) of music are played in motion picture and television sound tracks? Why? Walk into a gambling casino. What type(s) of music are played? Why?

A natural environment fosters healing. An artificial environment fosters devolution.

Music and sound. Refer to Section #21 for a discussion on the role of music in healing. Be aware of the sounds and noises in your environment and their impact upon stress and health.

Organization and structure. As explained in Section #13, one function of the brain helps the human to make sense of his/her environment. An inherent sense of organization and order must be perceived by the brain; otherwise we could not handle the sense of chaos. Organization, order, and structure imply a sense of control. This is important for stress management (Section #18) as well as for the left brain cognitive processor (Section #9). For example, I trust that the chair I am sitting on is not going to defy the law of gravity. I trust that my car is going to start and get to my business appointment, that I will arrive and return home safely and not be carjacked while on the road. I anticipate that my home will not have burnt down while away. A sense of control, order and organization is critical for the individual.

The person returning home from the hospital has just been through an uncontrolled and chaotic crisis. Just because the stress occurred in the past does not mean the recall (memory) of the crisis and all the emotions connected with it are also in the past. The recall and concomitant emotions are still occurring. Consequently, while still continuing the process of physically healing, the person is literally needing something of a return to normalcy. What can be done to help the co-therapist experience some of the normal routine?

A left brain cognitive processor naturally needs structure in his/her life, including the environment. A right brain cognitive processor (Section #9) is sensitive to environmental stimuli. In addition to routine normalcy items, be aware of clutter and signs of disorganization. As folks in Lancaster County, PA, say, "redd up the room." (Straighten up that room.) In addition, routine and structure are critical to a person experiencing senile dementia, such as Alzheimer's Disease.

Color. Use appropriate color schemes, if possible, in the healing environment. Some of the colors and their connotations for healing are as follows (Ref. #10):

- Blue: mental authority; relaxation (especially dark blue)
- Green: healing; reduction of nervous and muscular tension. Green also associates with nature's flow. Green or colors such as periwinkle blue (blue and green) are used in surgical areas to overcome glare (the stark contrast produced by white walls and body tissue for example) and relax the eyes. These colors compliment the red hue of body fluid and blood. This was how this color became to be associated with healing (Ref. #72)
- Yellow: cheerfulness and stimulation
- Brown: physical sensory association; familiar security; roots and the hearth. Subliminally, browns, beiges, and the spectrum of earth tone colors convey a "trust me" message
- Peach and Rose: warmth; enhancement of spiritual will to heal

2. Increasing the Quality of Social Support

This component of a home healing environment consists of many factors. Three major ones are discussed here:

- The importance of relaxation for the caregiver and the co-therapist
- Education and training
- The importance of touch

The importance of relaxation for the caregiver and the co-therapist. Recall from Section #19 the three-stage "General Adaptation Syndrome." In a time of crisis, the body cannot indefinitely sustain its energy. Long-term chronic stress impairs health and suppresses the immune system. Hence it is important for the caregiver to do such things as:

- Plan, develop and establish the physical home healing environment before the co-therapist arrives home from the hospital
- Recognize that the home healing environment is as important to the caregiver's stress level as it is to facilitating healing for the co-therapist
- Actively engage in and utilize the self-health tools found in this book and those listed in the Resources and Bibliography sections (#31 and #32)

Education and training. Recall from Section #24 that patient education is classified as social support.

An adult loses 80 percent of newly learned information within the next 24 hours (Ref. #18) - under normal conditions. Experiencing a healthcare crisis is stressful to everyone concerned. As stress increases, the ability to recall new, learned knowledge and skills decreases (Ref. #103).

It is vitally important for both the caregiver and the co-therapist to know and understand how to operate any home health equipment; how to perform prescribed treatments; to know their medication schedule; and how to follow special diets. Each of us, when we become a patient or a caregiver, has these responsibilities. Some of the practical things we can do to aid ourselves are these:

- Request, as a part of your patient rights to understand treatment, that you be allowed to tape the instructions in order that you may understand and remember them, especially if you have visual problems
- Ask for written counseling instructions regarding medication, side effects, foods to avoid, and other information deemed pertinent to the recovery process
- Ask for all pertinent educational materials. These help serve as a reinforcer of learning. Ask for actual on-the-job training in any special equipment. Do not allow the therapist/trainer to leave the room until both of you are satisfied that you know how to use the equipment. This implies practice and involves demonstration and return demonstration of taught skills, step-by-step
- If you are an older adult learner (age 40 and above), some special considerations (physiological and mental) impede the learning process (Ref. #103). These are reduced psychomotor responses leading to lower reaction time and slower assimilation of new material. An older learner needs to learn at his/her own pace. Demand that you be allowed to work at yours

Because of the crisis being experienced by the co-therapist, the caregiver must help ensure that both of you know and understand the education and training necessary for facilitating the healing process.

The importance of touch. As Ornstein and Sobel report (Ref. #82), we Americans are a maze of contradictions where touch is concerned. Our language contains elements of touch, but that's where it stops. These studies show that we touch much less than other cultures. It is as if our language attempts to compensate for lack of physical and emotional touching.

We use expressions such as "rub us the wrong way." "Be in touch." "I'm touched by..." Woe be to the aspiring bureaucrat or politician who has "lost touch." We're so out of touch with our feelings that we even have, as discussed above (see "Natural environment"), words like buttons and switches as metaphors for feelings. The reader can think of more.

Perhaps language needs to compensate because of our fear of touch due to political correctness; sexually transmitted diseases and the scourge of AIDS; fear of being labeled a child abuser; fear of being charged with sexual harassment, etc.

But touch is needed for health and human development - from maternal nurturing and touching as a matter of policy in premature infant wards through offering *therapeutic touch* in healthcare settings. (For a description of Therapeutic Touch, see Appendix A.) Sex, encompassing all the senses on the conscious level, is a touching experience, literally and figuratively. Touching physically is also a way of expressing feelings.

Touching bridges the isolation and fear experienced by the co-therapist. For example, at home the co-therapist may not be feeling particularly sexy with a catheter, but touch is still possible and needed. Touch can help alleviate those times when the significant other as caregiver and the co-therapist get on each other's nerves. There is a whole range of choice between physical isolation and sexual union culminating in orgasm. Touch bridges the duality between all or nothing. In addition to the "significant other", other caregivers - such as family or friends - can provide social support through touch.

However, for some people, due to past experiences or personality factors, touch is not therapeutic. Caregivers and supportive friends must be sensitive to the needs of these people.

3. Incorporating Stress Management and Wellness

(For review of these topics, refer to Section #18).

The co-therapist, in addition to the caregiver(s), as described above, has responsibility for treating not only the disease by following prescribed treatment regimen but also the illness accompanying the disease. He/she, as much as possible, should implement appropriate stress management strategies. Some alternatives have been recommended in this book.

Recall from Section #18 that the three components of hardiness are challenge, control and commitment. The co-therapist could be using this recovery time to examine any life style behaviors that may have contributed to the disease. As explained in Section #7, this must be done without engaging in "blaming the victim" games. The co-therapist could be using this time to ascertain how to regain meaning in his/her life.

Both the co-therapist and caregiver must recognize the inherent stress in the recovery period and communicate their needs to each other. No one is a mind reader. Feelings and demands should be allowed to be emotionally expressed without guilt being felt by either party. Both parties need to assist each other in making implicit assumptions explicit. For example, given the fact that Miles T. Gogh has always been a social extrovert, Martha M. Marvel-Gogh assumes that her husband, Miles, would love to have his golfing buddies and friends at work, especially his wonderful boss Mr. Styne, visit him frequently. Upon the day of discharge, Miles assumes that Martha knows he is in no mood to see anybody, especially his obnoxious boss, Franklin L. Styne.

Making explicit that which is implicit should be done as soon as possible, even prior to discharge. Assisting each other to reveal the hidden assumptions becomes part of the communications contract between the cotherapist and the caregiver.

Footnotes: (1) The American Academy of Pediatrics has cited over 1000 studies that positively link street violence to screen violence. This mega research was summarized in Bill Hendrick, "Violent TV, films are harming kids, pediatricians say" Mind and Body Section, The Atlanta Constitution, Wed., June 16, 1996.

References: 3, 10, 18, 72, 82, 103, 108

#26: IMAGERY AND HEALING

Definition and Characteristics

Imagery can be defined as multisensory integration.

Exercise: On a piece of paper, list the number of senses you have. When you complete your answer, continue reading. After reading this subsection, compare the number listed here with your recorded number.

The conscious sensory stimuli number six. These are:

- Seeing
- Hearing
- Touching
- Tasting
- Smelling
- Motion

Consciousness is immediacy. Feel the clothes you are wearing. Hear the sounds in your environment about you as you read this sentence. You are seeing these words as you read them. If you're smoking, eating, or drinking, experience the taste. What aromas, smells are in your environment? Feel yourself move; be aware of your bodily movements as you breathe.

These same six senses exist in the mental realm as well. They are used when we fantasize, day dream, and think. Right now, don't even think of a pink elephant. What comes to your mind? Imagine yourself sucking a raw lemon. What physical sensations come to you? Imagine yourself making love with your significant other. What senses do you experience? Think of your favorite sport or hobby. Do you see, in your mind, the words that spell out your favorite sport or hobby, or do pictures and other senses come to your mind?

The senses also exist in the subconscious realm. Do you dream? Do you see things in your dreams? Do you hear in your dreams? Is there a sense of movement in your dreams? You may even be able to experience smell or taste in your dreams.

Finally, a sense of clairsentience or extra sensory perception (ESP), can be developed. ESP occurs when you feel someone is watching you and you look around as the other quickly looks away. Have you ever felt a specific person, for no apparent reason, is going to call you? Then the phone rings and that person is the caller. Others have well-developed gifts of premonition, either for positive or negative events.

Thus, each person has three levels (physical, mental, and subconscious) of six senses each. Furthermore, many of us have also experienced at one time or another the ability of ESP. Hence we have 19 senses.

Sensory integration takes place in the limbic system (Section #16). Thus there is direct linkage between the use of imagery in stress management, healing, relaxation training, and learning.

Clinical Research

In the 1970s, O. Carl Simonton, a radiation oncologist, and Stephanie Simonton, a psychologist, received publicity for their work in teaching cancer patients how to use imagery to fight cancer. The Simontons reported an increase in longevity among the patients with whom they worked (Ref. #100). In the last two decades, no definitive, well researched cluster of studies has been done to prove whether this technique improves the statistical odds for survival for those with cancer (Ref. #48, Chapter 17).

However, research studies do definitely indicate that the use of imagery may help treat various physical maladies due to the relaxation response (Section #18) that imagery can help invoke. These ailments treated by imagery and relaxation include (Ref. #48, Chapter 17):

- Chronic pain
- Allergies
- Colds and flu
- Strains and sprains
- Stress-related ailments, such as hypertension and gastrointestinal problems

The most common application of imagery in healthcare application is the latter: stress reduction via relaxation training (Ref. #48, Chapter 17).

Proper Use of Imagery in Healing

Swartz has utilized imagery in his training classes involving accelerated learning and stress management, and in counseling for the last 12 years. For imagery to work most effectively, the following points are given for both the lay person and the healthcare professional:

1. Imagery is NOT visualization. Far too many counselors and stress management consultants confuse visualization with imagery. Many have told Swartz it is just semantics. Wrong. First of all, 40 percent of the population cannot visualize (Ref. #95). They may hear. They may feel. But they can't visualize. Visualization is seeing. Seeing is but one of the 19 senses that we possess.

Furthermore, the term *visualize* has important connotations. It is being divorced, separated, apart from the object for which you are striving . If I say to you, "Visualize yourself in your favorite place of relaxation (such as a beach)," you might interpret this request as seeing yourself sitting on a beach, just as you would view a home movie of yourself. But are you feeling the sand, smelling the salty air, tasting the lemonade made in the cooler, hearing the surf, aware of the movement of gulls?

Healing is defined as a movement toward wholeness (Section #5); wellness is being in the movement towards wholeness. *Being* implies active participation. *Visualization*, the way it is often practiced and the way many people are unfortunately trained, is passive and detached.

For an example of the proper use of imagery, refer to the "Creating a Relaxation Sanctuary" exercise in Section #27.

If you are going to use imagery to fight cancer, you must be the white T cell (Section #15) eating or killing the infected cell. What do you see as you travel through your blood stream? What does eating a cancerous cell taste like? What do you hear? What sense of motion do you have? This does not need to be disgusting. Suspend your left brain judgment and let the innate body/mind intelligence (Section #13) do its work. For example, what are some of your favorite tastes? Substitute and experiment.

However, this does require you to be a co-therapist. You need to have some knowledge of how the disease works and how the immune system fights this disease (Section #15). This is your responsibility as the patient or co-therapist.

Educate yourself before practicing these techniques.

You may also use imagery to help avoid some of the side effects of medication and treatment. For example, Dr. Bernie Siegel reported that negative programming is one reason why 25 percent of patients regurgitate prior to receiving their next chemotherapy treatment (Ref. #99).

Accompanying beliefs and internal dialogue are images. Stop as you catch yourself saying something and ask yourself: What beliefs are involved? What images are conjured up in your mind?

You may wish to use imagery as medical treatment. Again, be the medical treatment and follow through as above. But know how the medical treatment fights the disease. This leads to another important point.

2. *Imagery is NOT a substitute for prescribed medical treatment.* From the above examples, it may *supplement* such treatment, but it is not a *substitute* for such treatment.

3. *To be effective in using imagery to supplement medical treatment, one must first of all be in a state of relaxation.* See Section #19 for the importance of relaxation to healing.

4. *The use of imagery is important to elicit the relaxation response.* Hence it is important for stress management (Section #18). Refer to the exercises found in Section #27 for methods used to elicit the relaxation response. For other methods, refer to Section #18, especially Table 1.

5. *Effective use of imagery involves use of appropriate music* (Section #21). Music evokes imagery, emotions, and memories - all functions of the limbic system (Section #16), which is instrumental in eliciting the relaxation response.

References (Sources cited in this section): 48, 95, 99, 100
References (Sources used as general reference works for this section): 1

#27 RELAXATION EXERCISES

The exercises offered here, developed by R. G. Swartz and Associates (Resources, Section #31), are extremely beneficial to stress management, healing, and learning because they foster the relaxation response. (Sections #18; #26; and "Accelerated learning as training methodology", Section #10, respectively.)

The author strongly recommends that you, the reader, study this complete section before practicing any of the exercises.

Exercise I: "Creating a Relaxation Sanctuary"

This exercise is intended to create a mental place of relaxation, by using both physical and imaginative (sensory) means. The steps of the exercise follow:
(1) Play appropriate background music (Section #21) during the exercise. Kobialka's *Timeless Motion,* an Alternative Music composition (Section #30, Appendix C), is strongly recommended.
(2) As the music plays, decide on a relaxation sanctuary that you would find appealing (i.e., the most relaxing place and situation you can imagine); write a description of this place, placing it at the top center of a piece of unlined paper.
(3) On the same page, below and to the right, list the six senses:

TASTE
HEARING
SMELL
TOUCH
VISION
MOTION

(On your paper, leave space between each listed sense.)
(4) Next to each sense, on the left side of the page, list a few key descriptive words and/or phrases to indicate how you would use each sense in your relaxation sanctuary. Use present tense language. The subconscious and the brain's right hemisphere (Section #9) work with timelessness: the eternal now.
(5) Create mental images for the descriptions listed. If desired, note the images on the same page (Section #11, particularly the "Left/Right Note Study System").
(6) Take a few deep breaths and close your eyes. Recall your relaxation sanctuary and as many of your mental images as possible. (You may wish to combine this

exercise with the following by utilizing diaphragmatic breathing in place of a few deep breaths.)

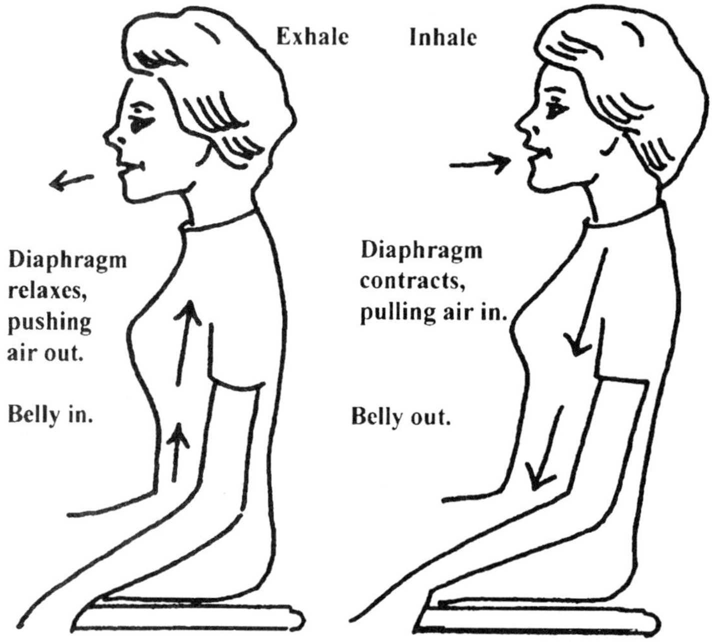

Figure 27.1 Diaphragmatic Breathing

Exercise II : The "22 Count" Breathing Exercise

The purpose of this exercise is to create a balanced relaxed, yet alert state, the optimal state for learning and healing. It also offers practice in abdominal breathing (see below) and can be done in combination with Exercise I.

Preparation. You are advised to read all instructions before beginning this exercise. To prepare for the exercise:
(1) During the exercise, play appropriate background music, such as Kobialka's *Timeless Motion* or *Dream Passage* (Section #30, Appendix C) or recordings of environmental sounds that are associated with your relaxation sanctuary .
(2) Sit comfortably on a chair or sofa or on the floor. Do not lie on the floor; doing so may cause you to become drowsy and lose mental focus. Why? Any appropriate relaxation technique and meditation properly done may create increased energy. The body, drained of energy, now experiences energy flowing through it. It's a "cultural shock" for the body. Drowsiness and sleep may thus

result. The goal of this exercise is to create a relaxed, yet alert state; sleep negates that goal.
(3) Loosen and/or remove your tie, constricting jewelry, and shoes. Place your feet flat on the floor (if you are sitting on a chair or sofa). Rest your hands, palms up, on your thighs.
(4) Become aware of your body touching the surface on which you are sitting and of your clothing touching your body; this awareness is called *focusing* or *centering*. The position of your body should manifest the self-centering that occurs mentally and emotionally within it (this is the true meaning of self-centeredness).

Diaphragmatic Breathing. The body's heart rate, blood pressure, and breathing rate involuntarily synchronize with musical rhythms, creating alpha brain wave states that produce the relaxation response, diminish stress, promote healing, and enhance learning (Section #19). Playing appropriate music during breathing exercises aids in the achievement of targeted breathing and heart rates (Section #21).

Rhythmic breathing is key to relaxation training and accelerated learning; the key to rhythmic breathing is diaphragmatic (abdominal) breathing.

The diaphragm, a large muscle situated just below the lungs, separates the lungs from the abdominal cavity. When inhaling, the stomach pushes outward and the diaphragm contracts, pulling air into the lungs (Figure 27.1). When exhaling, the stomach falls inward and the diaphragm is relaxed, pushing air out of the lungs (Figure 27.1). This synchronization is established by the deep sigh that initiates the diaphragmatic breathing exercise. Diaphragmatic breathing provides the brain with increased oxygen (i.e., at least eight times the volume of chest inhalations, which provide approximately 500 centimeters of air), giving the body more energy. It also fosters relaxation and health (Ref. #14).

Dr. Joan Borysenko, former director of Mind/ Body Clinic of Boston's Beth Israel Hospital and instructor of medicine at Harvard Medical School (Section #31), describes the steps of diaphragmatic breathing (Ref. #14):
(1) Sit comfortably, become self-centered, and place one hand on the stomach.
(2) Sigh deeply through your mouth, feeling the stomach fall in slightly; gently contract the stomach muscles slightly to exhale the last bit of air.
(3) With your hand still on your stomach, close your mouth and inhale through your nose, feeling the stomach expand. If the abdomen remains flat, you are breathing from your chest rather than your diaphragm; if this is the case, repeat steps 2 and 3, this time using the stomach muscles to push outward.

(4) Feel the stomach extend as the lower and upper portions of your lungs fill with air.
(5) Exhale through your nose, emptying the lungs and diaphragm; slightly contract the stomach muscles if necessary.
(6) Feel the abdomen fall as air leaves your lungs.
(7) Continue breathing in this manner, feeling your abdomen rise and fall, your shoulders move up and down, and your body rock slightly.
(8) Breathe normally; continue your activities.

Performing the "22-Count" Breathing Exercise. You are encouraged to use diaphragmatic breathing in the 22-count breathing exercise. The steps of the exercise follow:
(1) Play appropriate music during the exercise (Section #21). Dim or turn off artificial lighting.
(2) Sit comfortably in the study area (the established learning environment).
(3) Become self-centered; recall your relaxation sanctuary and the mental (sensory) images you created for it to assist you in becoming self-centered.
(4) Inhale abdominally, holding your breath for 22 counts (counting slowly) or as many counts as feel comfortable to you.
(5) Exhale.
(6) Repeat steps 4 and 5 two more times.
(7) Close your eyes and breathe normally.
(8) Imagine yourself in your relaxation sanctuary; try to feel as many of the senses associated with it as possible.
(9) Slowly return your thoughts to the reality of your environment. Wiggle your fingertips and toes, stretch your arms and legs, and feel the surface you are sitting on, the clothes you are wearing, and the floor your feet are touching. Become aware of the sounds of your environment.
(10) Open your eyes slowly. Stand and stretch.

Additional Notes for the 22-Count Breathing Exercise. You may wish to play subliminal tapes with messages that approximate the intent of the 22-count breathing exercise while performing the exercise, or to record and play your own audio cassette of the steps of the 22-count breathing exercise. The tape is more effective if the narrative is recorded in your own voice; this reinforces your taking responsibility for your relaxation, learning and healing.

(For guide lines for the consumer as to what constitutes an effective subliminal tape - both in terms of message wording and technical production - the reader is urged to consult Ref. #103, especially Section #14 of this reference.)

During the exercise, you are encouraged to allow your thoughts to flow without inhibition or interruption. The objective is to slow the thought process (aided by the slow, rhythmic cadence used in counting to 22) but still allow a free flow of thoughts.

Attempting to force an emptying of the mind of all thoughts is not encouraged. Because such a mental state is difficult to attain, the attempt to achieve it often causes the very tension that you are trying to relieve.

For the same reasons, forcing relaxation is also discouraged. After failing at forced relaxation, people may become frustrated and experience guilt feelings when considering the reasons for their failure. This increases rather than relieves anxiety.

To avoid such frustrations and tension-creating situations, Swartz recommends that you focus on breathing exercises and such exercises as the creation of a relaxation sanctuary. These are activities that foster comfortable, stress-free learning and healing environments.

Physiological Effects of Relaxation Exercises

Many individuals initially experience a few negative side effects of relaxation exercises, including:

- *Temporary swelling of the fingers*. This results from increased energy in the body and will subside soon after exercises are completed. Participants may wish to remove rings before beginning exercises
- *Tingling or twitching of arms and/or legs*. This is due to a release of pent-up energy
- *Slight tension or headache*. These effects may occur in those for whom focusing on relaxation:
    - Is an "in-tense" challenge. Some individuals force their eyes closed while concentrating on relaxing. This can cause physical strain and tension that can result in headaches
    - Creates anxiety and/or fear. Lower limbic, left dominant information processors and learners (Section #9) are especially apprehensive about risk taking or making changes in learning styles
    - Is so strange to them that the body reacts to the increased energy surge created by the relaxation exercises. The brain creates

energy; the body is electric (Ref. #103)

To aid relaxation, learners may wish to repeat the following sets of affirmations prior to exercise:

- I am relaxed yet alert
- I am feeling refreshed and at peace
- I am free of tension
- I am free of negative thoughts and feelings
- I am relaxation being
- I am harmony being
- I am easement being
- I am physical health being
- I am mental and emotional health being
- I am relaxed

Professional Assistance

Participants desiring advanced training in relaxation therapies (e.g., meditation and yoga - Section #18) are encouraged to seek assistance from qualified professionals rather than attempt to learn these therapies on their own. As with all accelerated learning/healing methods, such therapies are intended to supplement rather than substitute for medical treatment regimens. Refer also to appropriate resources listed in Section #31.

References: 14, 103

#28: PHYSICAL EXERCISE

NOTE: If you are older than 40 and/or have a physical ailment, consult with your physician before beginning any physical exercise program or any physical exercise.

The Need

When we look back on our ancestors who moved from their native countries and developed our country, we find these pioneers facing hard working, physically demanding challenges. Without cars to transport them, they either walked or used horses to transport them to their destination. Their lives were far more physically challenging than ours. We have become a sedentary society and seem to like it that way.

More than 40 medical studies have found that physically inactive people have approximately twice the number of heart attacks and heart disease as physically active people (Ref. #82). This life style behavior, popularly known as the "couch potato," involves as much risk as cigarette, cigar, and pipe smoking.

Physical exercise in moderate amounts is good for all people, no matter what stage of health they are experiencing. The key is to determine, with guidance, how much exercise is good for you and what your limitations are. Working within your limitations to stretch yourself physically is one of the best things you can do for yourself.

Physical Benefits of Exercise

When co-author Peske orients new patients to her rehabilitation center for pulmonary therapy, they look at her treadmills with terror and awe. She knows what they are thinking: "You mean I'd do that? No way. Not for me." When she explains, when she continues to empathize, that anyone and all people can learn how to exercise; that she'll be with them as they do it; that they can do it, she can see the glimmer of hope and belief in their eyes. She responds with: "Try it. You will see!"

Those professionals working in the clinical areas of rehabilitation appreciate the value of exercise. They see the physiological benefits of exercise as:

- Decreased arthritic pain

- Decreased blood pressure
- Weight reduction
- Increased muscle strength and tone
- Increased circulatory cardiac output (indirectly strengthening the cardiac muscle)
- Increased mental-physical balance
- Increased ventilation, challenging the respiratory system
- Smoother operating bowels
- Decreased appetite
- Control of anxiety

Physical exercise is also a means of eliciting the relaxation response (Section #18). Consequently, it is a stress management (Section #18) technique. Dr. Sacks (Ref. #48, Chapter 19) separates anxiety into two components; people, according to his studies, are prone to experience either one or both of these components:

- Cognitive, which is characterized by:
    - Mental anguish
    - Worrying
    - Irrational ideas
- Physical, which is the physiological reactions to stressors (for a definition, refer to Section #17) manifesting in the body

According to Sacks, those persons prone to experiencing the physical component may benefit best from physical exercise. However, just the fact of concentrating on something else, such as exercise, may also produce psychological benefits as well (see below).

Mental methods of invoking the relaxation response (imagery - Section #26; relaxation exercises - Section #27; meditation - Section #18; and Ref. #48, Chapter 15) may be best for those people prone to experiencing mainly emotional anxiety.

These are not hard and fast rules. As Sacks indicates, each person needs to experiment and find the best type of exercise and/or combinations that work for him/her.

One of the first reactions people have when they think about exercising is "I don't have enough energy now; how can I expend anymore energy for exercise?" When Peske teaches patients about energy, she always uses the cup of water analogy. She holds up an empty cup and says "Your source of energy will run dry if you don't fill it up on a regular basis. Just like this cup, which will empty if I don't continue to fill it up after I drink the water, so will my energy level become depleted if I don't decide how to fill it up." Pour out a little bit - fill up a little - use it - replenish it - the cup will remain full! The secret is to find out what you enjoy, what will stretch you to your limits. When you do it, you see your limits increase.

When a person begins an exercise program, the most significant body reaction will be one of fatigue. (To be honest, you might feel exhausted!) Even if a person begins slowly, as recommended, the body becomes aware of the change. Something is different. It takes a lot of motivation to keep on with the regimen because only after a month of this new routine does one begin to notice the physiological benefits from the life style change. The most critical time in the process is the first month of the new regime. People need to be encouraged to stick with it, because the body does adjust to increased activity. They will enjoy the benefits.

Psychological Benefits of Exercise

As an exercise enthusiast from way back, Peske has tried many types of exercise and has succeeded in some forms of regular exercise. She began her all-time favorite, aerobic dancing, 17 years ago when she was pregnant with her third child. She was experiencing emotional stress in her life and felt the need to enroll in a regular program. Physically, she was all right, but mentally she felt "stuffed up." Physiologically, she felt as if her insides were stagnant and like blood just recirculated through her body giving her little energy. She describes the feeling as being "crowded inside." Exercise for her became the relief she felt she needed: It stretched her. It increased her energy levels and convinced her of the need to adopt exercise as a lifetime behavior.

Psychological benefits of exercise generally include (Ref. #48, Chapter 19):

- Improved self-confidence
- Improved mood
- Feeling less depressed
- Obtaining and maintaining an increased energy level

Exercise offers a diversion. It is an outlet for the release of physical tension associated with the fight or flight response (Section #18). It is also a way of regaining an element of control in one's life. Recall from Section 18 that control is a major component in developing hardiness to stress. If exercise is done within a group setting, it becomes a means of socialization and a form of social support (Section #24).

What Types of Physical Exercise are Beneficial?

As a reaction to the country's laziness when it came to exercise and our sedentary life style, the American College of Sports Medicine in the 1970's issued a formula for fitness: 15-60 minutes of continuous exercise 3 to 5 times per week. This formula also called for exercise to be strenuous enough to raise the heart rate to 65 to 85 percent of the maximum (calculated as 220 minus the person's age). Millions of people began skiing, rowing, etc., joining health clubs to stand in line to use the equipment or its facilities. The goal? Bronzed versions of Adonis and Venus. "No pain, no gain" was burned into the nation's psyche. God is fitness.

A God who creates also destroys. A God who creates the Body Beautiful in the short term plants the seeds for self-destruction in the long term. Ornstein and Sobel (Ref. #82) present these statistics:

- 20 percent of all joggers who run 10 miles per week are injured severely enough to have to cut back on their exercise program
- 40 percent of those jogging more than 30 miles per week on pavement are injured severely enough to have to reduce their exercise program
- Injury rates soar for those working out strenuously every day - more than 30-45 minutes per session
- Strenuous levels of exercise can seriously disrupt women's reproductive systems
- Some women may not ovulate or they may miss their menstrual periods

More research is indicating this: gain yes, pain no. Ornstein and Sobel (Ref. #82) report major health gains with moderate exercise. A study of 12,000 middle-aged men indicated that those who burned 1600 calories a week had approximately 40 percent fewer heart attacks than those who burned fewer than 500 calories per week. 1600 calories burned in exercise equates to on-going leisure activities including:

- Walking a half-hour per day
- Gardening
- Dancing
- Participation in sports such as bowling, fishing or golfing

Those engaging in strenuous exercise, burning 4500 calories a week, did not as a group experience any additional decline in cardiac fatalities.

Ornstein and Sobel discovered that a long-term study of 17,000 Harvard alumni demonstrated that the healthy benefits of exercise (above) began for those burning up as few as 500 calories per week. This 500 calorie consumption equates to:

- A 15-minute walk per day
- 2 hours of bowling per week
- A one-hour game of squash

At this level (500 calories consumed with moderate exercise) death rates declined by 20 percent.

Hence, five words summarize this research: **continuous physical exercise in moderation.**

Special Factor: Chronic Disease

Exercise is essential for people who live with chronic disease. Chronic disease is draining. It affects all the physiological systems of the body. Stress in increased. The natural downward health spiral of the person experiencing a chronic disease can be negated when a person builds up his/her natural energy reserves. People living with chronic disease especially need to challenge their bodies through regular exercise at a pace that works for them in order to maintain the quality of life remaining.

However, before beginning any exercise regimen, it is important for the individual with chronic disease to follow these guide lines:

1. Visit your doctor first and discuss your intentions. Remember to recall your physical condition, including your chronic disease - especially if your physician is new.
2. In exercising, start out slowly.
3. If you are out walking, always leave enough energy to return home. The distance out is the same as the distance back.
4. Learn to take your pulse. Subtract your age from 220 (maximal heart rate). Take 65 percent of this sum; then take 95 percent of this sum. Keep your heart rate within this range.
5. Maintain your exercise programs for at least a month before you decide to quit due to fatigue. The fatigue should gradually decrease. If pain increases, stop and see your doctor. Monitor yourself.
6. Remember to give yourself credit. Appreciate your desire and determination to increase your energy level and stamina.
7. Go for it! Move your body and stretch yourself.

References: 48, 82

#29: NUTRITION

Overview

So much of what we currently read in the recent literature on life style behavior changes focuses on nutrition, defined as "the act or process of ... being nourished; the sum of the processes by which an animal or plant takes in and utilizes food substances" (Merriam Webster's Collegiate Dictionary, Tenth Edition, 1993).

Medical studies estimate that 40 percent of all cancers in men and 60 percent in women are related to diet (Ref. #71). Diet has been implicated in two major risk factors associated with coronary heart disease (CHA):

- High blood cholesterol
- Hypertension

Diet is of course a factor in being overweight, which itself contributes to CHA, and certain types of diabetes (Ref. #71). Diet can also play a role in preventive medicine and helps reverse atherosclerosis - hardening of the arteries (Ref. #24).

Nutrition involves responsibility not only for what types and amounts of foods we put into our bodies but paying attention to the substances those foods contain (see following subsection, "food substances"). Yet we, as healthcare consumers, often do not pay attention to either the medical reports or to the types and amounts of foods consumed.

We rush. We eat on the run. We virtually inhale our physical food, unaware of what we are eating. We don't cook for ourselves if we live alone; it takes too much time. We go out.

When our grandparents were children, all the family members worked, played and prayed hard. Most days were spent working in the fields, factory, or home. We think we work hard today! Our ancestors worked physically hard to till the soil, invent electricity and automobiles, and build cities, etc. At the end of every day, they met as families at the dinner table. Eating was not only a physical event but one including socialization and cultural and spiritual values. Eating together fulfilled many human needs besides the physical replacement of expended calories: needs for emotional, psychological, and spiritual development.

Think about our lives and the meals we share as families. More often, today, both parents work outside the home and there is little time for cooking. Many single people eat out, considering this more cost and time efficient. Families whip up dinner so adults can get on to meetings. We live, eat, socialize, and work in a hurry. No wonder we eat the wrong foods and in the wrong amount. How and when will we get this nutrition see-saw in balance? The body needs adequate nutrition of proper foods in adequate amounts in both health and sickness. The disease process of illness requires calories for healing. Tissue rejuvenation and replacement require foods to heal.

The United States is a land rich in milk and honey. Although the political and social problems of farmers and the homeless sometimes shadow our joy, most Americans have enough to eat. The amount of food we waste in our homes and restaurants would go far towards feeding the homeless. In fact, most of us probably eat more than we should most of the time. The reasons we eat include:

- Hunger
- Habit
- Emotional satisfaction
- Stress: both emotional and mental

Think of the body as made up of systems: physical, mental, emotional, and spiritual. We need to feed each one of these systems.

We are all aware of the physical foods which nourish us. The current trend of decreasing the fat intake in our diets to 10 percent is suggested by Dr. Dean Ornish (Ref. #48, Chapter 1) to decrease our personal risks of cardiac disease. (See also "fats and cholesterol", below.) Heart disease, our number one killer, occurs because we each have environmental, familial, and self-inflicted limitations. The self-limitation of lack of exercise coupled with overeating, or eating the wrong foods, places a person in severe jeopardy of developing, or furthering the development of, heart disease.

Heart disease is a slow, insidious process. You can't see the physical changes within your bodily system. You might experience warning signs of cholesterol levels, shortness of breath, angina-like chest pains, or high blood pressure but the usual reaction is one of conflict or denial. Then the heart attack occurs.

Cardiac catheterizations reveal blockages in the system of coronary vessels. Many times, the patient, although asymptomatic, has advanced disease. What has that person eaten all of his/her life? Are we "what we eat?"

Many of us eat too many calories and are overweight. The flip side of the coin holds the people who have eating disorders and are underweight. It is important for those of us in healthcare to be aware of our patients' eating problems. The nutrition departments at the hospitals have dietitians who help us and our patients with weight loss or gain. Those of us in nursing can help our patients with their nutritional problems by being aware, asking questions, and offering support in difficult situations.

Strict, calorie counting diets are not for everybody (see below). But we all should be aware of the value of the foods we put into our bodies. Some people feel that this knowledge of nutrition restricts their food choices too severely. Deleting the fats of eggs, bacon, butter and milk does limit breakfast choices, especially if you have traditionally eaten bacon and eggs. Foods have many preservatives and additives that are full of sodium and other chemicals causing cancer and hypertension. What can we eat? What is actually all right to eat?

Food Substances: Necessary Nutrients

As stated above, it is not the foods that directly contribute to the acquisition or prevention of disease, but rather the substances found in the foods. There are three major types of these substances, termed *nutrients*:

- Water
- Micronutrients
- Macronutrients

Water. The purpose of water is to provide fluid for chemical reactions (Section #13), circulation of blood, waste removal, and maintenance and regulation of body temperature. The body needs to replace two to three quarts of water per day (Ref. #71).

Micronutrients. Micronutrients consist of:

- Vitamins
- Minerals

The purpose of vitamins is to regulate chemical processes taking place in the body (Section #13). Minerals assist with chemical regulation and play a role in body maintenance in terms of forming new body tissue, bones, teeth, and blood. There have been many important discoveries on the necessity of vitamins and minerals for the maintenance of health, especially in the presence of illness and disease. If you have any chronic condition, such as coronary artery disease or diabetes, or are thinking of becoming pregnant, ask your doctor for specific information on supplements that would help you. (For additional information on vitamins and minerals, see Ref. #71 as well as "Additional Reading" at the end of this section.)

Macronutrients. The purpose of macronutrients is to provide energy for maintenance and repair of the body, and for physical growth. Macronutrients consist of:

- Carbohydrates
- Fats
- Protein

The body produces energy, a function of the macronutrients. The potential of any food to supply energy is measured in *calories. Carbohydrates* (below) provide 46 to 50 percent of the body's energy needs. One gram of carbohydrates equals four calories. Carbohydrates are an efficient fuel because they can provide energy almost immediately. *Fats* (below), including fat stored in the body, provide energy but not as efficiently as carbohydrates. One gram of fat equals nine calories. *Proteins* (below) are the body's basic building materials, necessary for growth and all bodily functions. One gram of protein equals four calories. 12 to 15 percent of our daily intake in calories should consist of proteins (Ref. #71).

The following statements need to be emphasized in any discussion concerning macronutrients (Ref. #71):

- The body begins to rely more on fats than carbohydrates for energy after approximately 20 to 30 minutes of continuous activity
- The longer a person goes without food, the more his/her body relies on fat for energy
- Any dietary fat consumed in food not burned by the body is converted into body fat

Elements of a Healthy Diet: the Basics

The following discussion summarizes major studies and guidelines formulated by the American Heart Association, the National Institutes of Health, and the National Academy of Sciences (Ref. #71). Two essential rules for obtaining a healthy diet are:

- *Avoid foods high in sodium, refined sugar, fats and cholesterol*
- Consume foods high in complex carbohydrates

Avoid foods high in sodium, refined sugar, fats and cholesterol. Daily intake of sodium, a needed mineral, should be no more than 2400 milligrams. This equates to one teaspoon of salt. High levels of consumed sodium, via salt, contribute to:

- Heart attack
- Stroke
- Kidney disease

Regarding the use of sugar, you should know that many foods high in sugar are also high in fat. Refined sugar and all sugars are simple carbohydrates.
For fats and cholesterol, the total daily intake of fats should be no more than 30 percent of the total number of calories consumed. Saturated fats should be no more than 10 percent of total calories (Ref. #71), because they contribute to high cholesterol levels.

Sources for saturated fats are:
- Dairy products, including butter, eggs, etc.
- Coconut and palm oil; vegetable oils
- Meats

A diet high in cholesterol contributes to heart disease. Cholesterol circulates in the blood. Accumulating in the walls of blood vessels as unused nutrients, it is referred to as plaque. Build-up of plaque contributes to atherosclerosis or hardening of the arteries. This, in turn, can contribute to heart disease, leading to heart attack or stroke (Ref. #71). For the relationship between stress and cholesterol, see Ref. #8. For the relationship between hostility and cholesterol, see Ref. #48, Chapter 4. In essence, both stress and hostility contribute to the build-up of plaque.

Cholesterol is not an essential, needed nutrient in terms of its being externally consumed into the body by foods. The cholesterol needed by the body is manufactured in the body by the liver.

There are two types of cholesterol having direct impact on blood cholesterol levels (Refs. #71 and #97):
- High Density Lipoproteins (HDL): good cholesterol
- Low Density Lipoproteins (LDL): bad cholesterol

LDLs, produced by saturated fats, raise blood cholesterol levels. Polyunsaturated fats tend to lower the amount of LDLs. Sources of polyunsaturated fats are corn, safflower and sesame oils. Sources of other unsaturated fats are plants and fish. However, it is important to know that large intakes of polyunsaturated fats have been implicated in development of some types of cancer (Ref. #71).

HDLs are known as the good cholesterol because they pick up cholesterol circulating in the blood vessels and return it to the liver for reprocessing or excretion. Reduction of saturated fats in the diet does not seem to affect the level of HDL cholesterol. A person cannot eat/consume good cholesterol (Ref. #71). Instead, HDLs can be raised to significant levels by stopping smoking, physically exercising more (Section #28), and losing excess weight (Ref. #97).

To determine the total calories of fat in a food, look at the label's contents. Find the number of grams of fat per serving. This will be listed on the label. Multiply this total by nine (the number of calories contained in one gram of fat).

Consume foods high in carbohydrates. There are two types of carbohydrates: simple and complex.

Simple carbohydrates are the sugars. There are various types of sugars. Refined white table sugar (sucrose) is derived from beets or sugar cane and refined. Other sugars are fructose, glucose, dextrose, etc.

Complex carbohydrates are the starches. Major sources of these carbohydrates are whole grains, rice, pasta, vegetables such as potatoes and beans, and fruits. Foods high in complex carbohydrates also contain supplemental nutrients such as vitamins, minerals, water, and fiber. Medical studies have found that dietary fiber is needed in prevention of heart disease, colon cancer, rectal cancer, diverticulitis, diabetes, breast cancer, and obesity (Ref. #71).

Recall that one of the two basic rules for a healthy diet is to consume foods rich in complex carbohydrates. Foods containing these supply a better balance of nutrients and are less fattening. Simple and complex carbohydrates contain four calories per gram as compared to nine calories per gram of fat.

For example, rich desserts are not fattening because they contain starch and sugar but because they are loaded with fat. At least 55 percent of our daily intake of calories should consist of complex carbohydrates (Ref. #71).

Protein

Protein constitutes 75 percent of the body's tissue, including the enzymes, or compounds that direct chemical reactions. (Refer to peptides and neuropeptides in Section #13.) The body uses protein to grow and to maintain and repair itself.

In the body, protein consists of 22 amino acids. Of the 22 known amino acids, the body itself can manufacture only 13; nine have to come from outside. Hence the importance of proteins to our diet. We can get them from plants (which manufacture internally all the amino acids required for their survival) or from animals that consume plants (Ref. #71).

Sources of these needed amino acids/protein are:

- Meat
- Fish
- Poultry
- Vegetables
- Dairy products
- Legumes
- Whole grains

However, remember to consume those sources that are lower in saturated fats. Go light on meats and dairy products, heavy on vegetables and whole grain.

References: 8, 24, 48, 71, 97

Additional Reading: For detailed information on the micronutrients, including vitamins and minerals, see Jean Carper, *Jean Carper's Total Nutrition Guide* (Bantam: NY), 1987; see also Ref. #31.

Resources: Refer to "Preventive Medicine Research Institute", Section #31, for Dr. Ornish's program for reducing the effects of atherosclerosis using nutrition.

SOURCE MATERIALS

Notes

Appendix A: ALTERNATIVE MEDICINE AND THERAPIES

Note: Those of the following preceded by an asterisk have received greater recognition by traditional medicine.

Some useful Internet addresses are included in the text and at the end of this section. If you do not have direct access to the Internet, your local library can access the information for you.

Acupressure
Stimulation of energy centers of the body with pressure (the same centers used for the needles in acupuncture) to promote healing. Electricity may be used instead of needles. Acupressure Institute (415) 845-1059.

Acupuncture
Chinese modality which stimulates the body's ability to sustain and balance itself through the use of sterilized needles at points on energy meridians. The premise: The body is a bioelectric system. This energy is called chi or qi (pronounced chee). When the natural flow is halted, pain and disease occur. Stimulating particular points on the skin with needles or heat rebalances the energy flow.

Approximately 2,000-3,000 doctors in the US use this method. Licensed by 21 states; in 24 states only certified physicians may perform this therapy. It has been shown to be effective in relieving arthritis and chronic pain as well as the stress created by trying to give up an addictive habit. As of 1992, 240,000 treatments per week were conducted. To find a licensed acupuncturist, contact: American Acupuncture Council (800) 838-0383 or http://www.acupuncture.com

Affirmation
Repeating a positive statement using the present tense. For examples, see "Physiological Effects of Relaxation Exercises," Section #27; see Section #13, Ref. #103, on how to properly word affirmations.

Alexander Technique
A type of body work which does not treat specific symptoms but facilitates the improvement of posture or carriage to help alleviate stress related illnesses, muscle tension and pain. Practitioners further postulate that a series of at least 10 sessions can help alleviate stress and stress related conditions such as depression, tension headaches, ulcers, exhaustion, asthma, respiratory problems, digestive problems, etc. N. American Society of Teachers of the Alexander Technique,

(217) 359-3529 or http://www.life.uiuc.edu/jeff/alextech.html

Aromatherapy
The art and controlled external use of pure essential oils distilled from aromatic plants to enhance health and beauty. Essential oils have a rejuvenating and balancing effect on the mind and emotions. Because senses are integrated in the limbic system (Section #16), there is direct clinical evidence for the interrelationship of scents, memories, and emotions. The most useful application of this therapy is stress management and learning rather than the direct cure of physical disease. For example, the sense of smell can trigger a wealth of memories and emotions connected to smell. Remember Vicks' salve?

According to Jean Valnet, M.D., a French doctor who utilized aromatherapy as medicine, there are oils that are antibacterial, etc., useful for treating many diseases.

Astrology
Study and application of influences of the stars and planets upon the lives of individuals. American Federation of Astrologers, P.O. Box 22040, Tempe, AZ 85285.

Ayurvedic Medicine (traditional Indian)
The Indian (Asian) tradition of the application of nutrition, meditation and herbs to physiological disease is thousands of years old. A popular proponent of such practice is Dr. Deepak Chopra, author of *Quantum Healing*.

The May, 1991, issue of the Journal of the American Medical Association ran a three page letter from Ayurvedic practitioners citing findings from various investigations. A plethora of research needs to be done.
Maharishi Ayurveda Association of America, P.O. Box 282, Fairfield, IA 52256 (515)472-8477.

Bach Flower Remedies
Floral essences used to relieve stress, for relaxation, etc. Dr. Edward Bach Healing Society, 644 Merrick Rd., Lynbrook, NY 11563 (516)593-2206.

***Biofeedback**
The science of using specially designed machinery to train clients how to control their seemingly uncontrollable body functions such as heart rate, blood pressure, and breathing for the purposes of relaxation. The equipment serves as instant feedback monitoring devices for the client so that the client can chart his/her progress (Ref. #48, Chapter 18).

***Chiropractic**
The science of claiming that health of the spine directly impacts the health of the physical body. It originated in this country in 1895 in Iowa. Misaligned vertebrae will cause malfunctions in the nervous system. Currently, chiropractic is the third largest primary healthcare profession in the Western hemisphere. Only medicine and dentistry outrank it. Some studies indicate that each year one in every 20 Americans sees a chiropractor. American Chiropractic Association (703)276-8800 or http://pages.prodigy.com/CT/doc/doc.html

Color Therapy/Healing
According to researchers, colors around us can dramatically alter moods. In general, bright warm colors provide energy while cool colors calm our emotions. This is based on the theory that the colors in light beams carry energy that is transmitted to us when we come in contact with them. People who do crystal healing/chakra healing/laying on of stones, etc., also use colors as part of their healing.

Crystal Healing
Using the earth energy of crystals to focus the energy of the body. The practitioner uses different crystals for different functions, to facilitate healing and/or physical cure. See books by Barbara Walker, Uma Silbey, Katrina Raphael and others for more information.

Dreamwork
Using dream interpretation for diagnosis and healing.

Faith Healing (laying on of hands)
Take up thy rug and walk. Many healing modalities use the laying on of hands approach to healing (Reiki, Therapeutic Touch, Massage Therapy, etc.).

Feldenkrais
A type of body work emphasizing movement and posture therapy which is designed to improve self-image, creativity and vitality. This therapy is based upon the ancient belief that the body is the mirror of the mind. The Feldenkrais Guild, POB 11145, San Francisco, CA 94101 (415)550-8708
or http://www.usc.edu/hsc/neuroprotection/feldenkrais/

Feng Shui
Chinese system of harmonious design of home or business for wealth, health and good fortune, i.e., adjusting environment through harmony.

Guided Imagery (Section #26)

Hellerwork
A system of deep tissue work. For more information, contact:
The Body of Knowledge (916)926-2500.

Herbal Medicine
This use of plants for healing is found in all world cultures. Preparations from plants are ingested. Practitioners claim their remedies contain natural ingredients that are as potent as synthetic drugs but safer, with fewer side effects. Several drug companies are currently doing research on medicinal properties of North American plants. American Herb Association, P.O. Box 99, Rescue, CA 95672. "Herbal Hall", a listing of resources: http://www.crl.com/~robbee/herbal.html

Holistic Healing
This medicine embraces the "Mind/body" connection and uses alternative as well as conventional treatments to promote healing. The focus is on the whole person rather than just the condition being treated:

American Holistic Medical Association (919)787-5146
American Holistic Nurses Association (same as above)
Holistic Dental Association (614)366-3309

Homeopathy
Developed by Samuel Hahnemann, a German doctor, in the 1800s, practitioners believe that symptoms such as fever should not be suppressed because they represent the body fighting the disease itself. Consequently, physical disease can be cured by using drugs that help the body. A person with a fever, for example, would be given a drug that would raise the fever. The administered doses are diluted. Not recommended for life threatening illnesses. Homeopathy cannot cure broken bones or vitamin deficiencies. National Center for Homeopathy. (202)223-6182 or http://antenna.nl:80/homeoweb/resources.html

***Hospice**
The concept of allowing a terminal patient with no possibility of physical cure to live the remainder of his/her life as fully as possible, using medications to relieve pain and assisting the patient and his/her family to deal with death and the concept of dying well. Hospice is available to anyone, regardless of income. In most cases, Medicare, Medicaid and private insurers cover most of their services to allow the patient to remain at home. National Hospice Organization (800) 658-8898.

***Hypnosis**
The process of using the inner self (Section #18 and Ref. #48, Chapter 16) as a healing tool to recover repressed and/or suppressed memories and the emotions connected to those memories that may be contributing to psychosomatic illness. Hypnosis is used either by the therapist, to give suggestions to the client, or by the client, to give suggestions to him/herself, if he/she is properly trained in this technique. American Institute of Hypnotherapy (714)261-6400.

Massage Therapy
Use of the hands to ease muscle soreness, drain toxins from the body, and create a state of relaxation. AMTA (American Massage Therapy Association) (847)864-0123.

Meditation (see "Prayer").
The art of developing spiritual awareness. (See also: Ref. #48, Chapter 15; Section #31, Stress Reduction Clinic)

Mental Healing (telepathic)
The conscious projection of healing energy upon another using mental imagery. The recipient of the energy may or may not be consciously aware of the intent of the other person(s). Another variation of this is the use of certain colors, such as mentally enveloping the person in brilliant white light. This is a New Age technique which, interestingly, relates to both spiritual prayer and the concept of telepathic communication.

***Music** (Section #21)
For an internet resource, check http://falcon.cc.ukans.edu/rment/mt.html

Naturopathy (natural medicine)
A doctor of naturopathy is not a medical doctor. American Association of Naturopathic Medicine (206)328-8510 or http://www.amrta.org/~amrta

***Nutrition** (Section #29)

***Osteopathy**
Developed in the late 1800s, this modality uses body manipulation to treat a variety of physical ailments. Osteopaths (DO's) are educated as thoroughly as medical doctors (MD's) and licensed with the same criteria. Unlike M.D.'s, their training consists of how to manipulate body tissue, joints and muscles to facilitate healing. American Osteopathic Association, 212 E. Ohio St., Chicago, IL 60611.

***Physical Exercise** (Section #28)

Polarity Therapy
According to Randolph Stone, the founder of polarity therapy, there is an electromagnetic field in all living things (an energy field). The energy field can be blocked by illness, stress, etc. Polarity therapy is the process of unblocking the energy field. American Polarity Therapy Association, POB 19459, Seattle, WA 98109.

Prayer
Prayer is talking to God. (Conversely, some people believe that meditation is God talking to you.) Prayer is going outside yourself, beyond physical boundaries. (Meditation is going inside to be silent, opening your higher self.) Truly religious prayer is premised upon this foundation: *Thy* will be done, not my will be done. *My* will be done is affirmation, not prayer.

Reflexology
Reflexologists claim that there are external points on the feet (and hands) representing every organ of the body. These points govern energy flow throughout the body. Through massage of these points, a practitioner can unblock blocked energy. International Institute of Reflexology (813)343-4811.

Reiki
A type of laying on of hands to balance energy. Reiki means universal life energy, called *ki* in Japan. Reiki originated in Tibet and was brought from Japan to the US in 1938. American International Reiki Association (213)394-6620.

***Relaxation Training**
Various modalities for the purpose of stress management programming. Sections #18, #19 and #27.

Rolfing
A system of body alignment exercises designed by Ida Rolf. Deep, painful massage is given to realign the body. The theory is no pain, no gain.
Rolf Institute, POB 1868, Boulder, CO 80306 (303)449-5903.

Shiatsu
Uses spinal manipulation and acupressure techniques. Uses physical pressure, not needles. Like acupressure, physical points are used which serve as channels of energy. The purpose of the therapist is to physically manipulate points along the spine which serve to unblock blocked energy channels, causing pain.

American Oriental Bodywork Therapy Association (609)782-1616.

***Stress Management** (Section #18)

Therapeutic Touch

This therapy is premised upon the existence of an energy sustaining all life. In China, this energy is chi or qi (pronounced chee). In India, it is known as prana. In physics, it is known as a force field. In a state of health this energy flows freely, balanced, and nourishes the body. The practitioner feels for the blockages and assists the client in releasing them.

Dr. Delores Kreiger helped popularize this technique in the early 1970's and introduced it to the professional schools of nursing, working with New York City hospitals. Documented positive results (accelerating the rate of healing) with this modality range from minor cuts and burns through recuperation from surgery. Advocates of this treatment report that results are independent of a patient's conscious beliefs as to the efficacy of this treatment.

Nurse Healers Professional Assoc., PO Box 444, Allison Park, PA 15101.

Trager

An innovative learning system of movement reeducation created and developed by Milton Trager, M.D. Utilizing gentle, nonintrusive movements, the Trager approach helps release deep-seated physical and mental patterns and facilitates deep relaxation, increased physical mobility and mental clarity. Currently, there are over 700 certified practitioners from 20 countries who practice in stress management centers, pain clinics, physicians' offices.

The Trager Institute (415)388-2688.

Vitamin Therapy

Dieticians and nutritionists will tell you that you should be able to get the vitamins you need, under normal circumstances, from your food. However, many doctors as well as nutritionists are using vitamin supplements to aid healing (the antioxidants Vitamin C, Vitamin E, Beta Carotene and the minerals Zinc and Selenium). This is part of nutritional therapy and research is beginning to show good results.

However, no medical doctor or dietician will approve unsupervised mega-vitamin therapy because some vitamins (A, D, and some of the B's) are toxic in large doses. Any mega-vitamin use should be closely monitored by a professional.

Also, diabetics and others need to know that mega-doses of Vitamin C will cause urine test results to be wrong, which could be dangerous to their health.

Yoga
A combination of stretching, breathing and meditation designed to yoke man to God, the physical to the spiritual. The practice of yoga keeps humanity's growth to God head in conscious awareness (Section #18 and Table 18.1. For the four major types of yoga, see Appendix D).

References: (Sources used as general reference works for this appendix): 7, 41, 89, 109.

Additional reading:

Harper's Encyclopedia of Mystical and Paranormal Experience. Harper Collins Publishers: NY, 1991.
New Age Sourcebook, 1991.
New Age Journal, Brighton, MA, 1991.
Peale, Norman Vincent. *The Power of Positive Thinking.* Prentice Hall:NY, 1952.
Stein, Diane. *All Women Are Healers: A Comprehensive Guide to Natural Healing.* 1990.
The World Almanac & Book of Facts. Scripps Howard:NY, 1991.
For information from the United States government on alternative medicine, contact: OAM Information Center, Office of Alternative Medicine, NIH, 6120 Executive Boulevard, EPS Suite 450, Rockville, M.D. 20892-9904 Telephone: 301-402-2466 FAX: 301-402-4741

Resources on the Internet:
If you have a commercial Internet provider, such as America Online, Compuserve, or Prodigy, there are many resources available - for example, on America Online, keyword "Health" to find information on both traditional and alternative medicine. You can search the internet through various on-line search services and data bases for information (AltaVista, Lycos, Yahoo, and Magellan are examples). Your local library can direct you to specific sites if you are not familiar or comfortable with "net surfing." A few interesting sites:

Allied and Alternative Medicine (AMED) is a commercial data base of complementary or alternative medicine: http://www.rs.ch/www/rs/ds/amed.html

The Alternative Medicine Homepage, which has links to many modalities mentioned in this appendix as well as other resources: http://www.pitt.edu/~cbw/altm.html

Medscape: the Online Resource for Better Patient Care, to find information on patient education: http://www.medscape.com

Therapeutics, which includes information on Osteopathic medicine, hypnosis and acupuncture: gopher://linux2.mic.ki.se/11/Biomed/Diseases/Therapeutics

World Wide Wellness: Internet Resources for Whole Living can be reached at: http://www.doubleclickd.com/wwwellness.html. Their directory of health professionals is listed at http://www.doubleclickd.com/directory.html

For anyone new to "net-surfing": it really is easy to do. You can do it on any computer with a modem, connected to an internet service. If you have a dinosaur with a 2400 baud modem, join America Online. Some of the direct connections require a fast modem and an up-dated computer system.

The internet sites listed were all active when this book went to the printer. However, due to the way the internet works, if someone up-dates their site, the URL (internet address) may change. To avoid the frustration of trying to remember the URLs, search for new information through AltaVista.

(On your Web browser - be it Netscape, AOL or other browser, type in: http://www.Altavista.digital.com and wait for it to load. AltaVista is the easiest search engine to use if you are interested in finding when information was posted, as it is all dated. Type in the subject you are looking for: for example, aromatherapy. AltaVista will give you a list of related sites, complete with a short description and the last date it was up-dated. All you do is "mouse-click" on the title of the site or its URL (internet address) and you will go directly to that site.

To get back to the list of sites after visiting one, merely click the "back" button on your browser and you will return to the list. (If you have visited several pages, you may have to click "back" several times to get back to the list.)

You can also search through other search engines, such as Yahoo, Lycos, etc. Just type in http://www.Yahoo.com or http://www.Lycos.com and go from there. You can send information to your printer directly from the internet or download it to read later, saving your online time.

Appendix B: BRAIN DOMINANCE OCCUPATIONAL PROFILES - NARRATIVE DESCRIPTIONS

The following narrative descriptions of representative healthcare professionals derive from assessment and interpretation of the Herrmann Brain Dominance Instrument (HBDI) as described in Section #9. Each represents the average, composite profile of the particular occupation. Each profile also represents the cognitive processing and learning style(s) of an individual associated with that given occupation.

Refer to Section #9 for an interpretation of each four-number heading below as well as for elaboration on cognitive processing and learning styles.

1-1-2-2: Hospital Administrator and Surgeon

This is a double dominant profile with primaries in the Left mode - Upper Left A and Lower Left B quadrants. It is the second most common profile in the general population, representing 15 percent, and the most common profile for males, representing 21 percent. The profile is characterized by a logical, analytic, technical orientation, and is effective in rational problem solving from the Upper Left A quadrant. Lower Left B quadrant preferences include planning, organizing, implementing and administrative activities. In this profile, the processing modes of Upper Left A and Lower Left B would clearly be the most preferred, and the interpersonal, emotional, and spiritual modes of Lower Right C and the holistic, creative, and synthesizing modes of Upper Right D would be at the secondary level, yet functional. This profile is typical of those occupations in technical fields, such as engineering and manufacturing, financial positions, middle managers, and in general, those positions for which left mode processing is clearly most important, and the right mode processing being necessary, yet secondary.

1-2-1-1: General Practitioner

This profile is triple dominant, with three preferred quadrants. These primaries occur in Upper Left A, Lower Right C, and Upper Right D quadrants. This is a multi-dominant profile that would be characterized by well balanced processing modes of Upper Left A - the analytic, logical, and rational processing; the interpersonal, emotional, and intuitive thinking modes of Lower Right C, combined with the artistic, creative, and holistic processing modes of the Upper Right D quadrant. The Lower Left B secondary quadrant would be functional, yet clearly of less preference in terms of organizing, control, structure and conservative thinking styles. This profile is also double dominant in the upper modes, both left and right. This individual would be more experimental than safe-keeping and more emotional than controlled. Occupations would involve those with less administrative detail and more attention to broad concepts, strategic planning as compared to operational planning, and those occupations tending towards a more "generalized" nature. Positions involving technical innovation and future planning fit this profile along with human resource and development professions.

2-1-1-1: Supervisory Nurse

This is a triple dominant profile with two primaries in the right mode, Lower Right C and Upper Right D quadrants, and the third in Lower Left B. It is the most common of all profiles, with 16 percent of the population exhibiting this multi-dominant array of preferences. It is the clear majority for the female population, 24 percent exhibiting this profile. The 2-1-1-1 profile is characterized by its multi-dominant and "generalized" nature, and fairly balanced amount of understanding and ability to use the three primary quadrants - the preferred processing modes being creative and holistic in Upper Right D, interpersonal and feeling in Lower Right C, and planning and organizing in the Lower Left B. The Upper Left quadrant A is least preferred, but still the person is typically quite functional in their use of the logical and analytical aspects of this quadrant. This profile is typical of many personnel and human resource professionals, including teachers as well as those whose occupations require an understanding and ability to function on many levels, such as social workers, executive secretaries, and supervisory nurses.

2-1-1-2: Nurse

This profile is a double dominant profile with the two primaries in the Lower Left B and Lower Right C quadrants. It is a double primary in the lower, visceral area. The profile is characterized by very strong preferences in conservative thinking and controlled behavior with a desire for organization and structure as well as detail and accuracy from the Lower Left B quadrant. Persons with this profile tend to worry about details. The primary in the Lower Right C would equally show itself by emotional and interpersonal preferences, an interest in music, and a sense of spirituality. It would also show in an intuitive "feelings" sense of this person. The two lower primaries could represent an important duality for the person to resolve within themselves. The opposing qualities of control and structure, of "form" - and the emotional and interpersonal "feelings" can cause internal conflict. The clear secondary preferences of the upper modes, both Upper Left A and Upper Right D, are also characteristic of this profile, with logical and analytical in the Upper Left A quadrant and holistic and creative thinking of Upper Right D quadrant. Occupations typical of those people with this profile include nurses, homemakers, secretaries, and other members of the "helping" profession.

2-2-1-1: Psychologist

This profile features two primaries in the right mode, quadrants C and D, and two secondaries in the left mode, quadrants A and B. It is the third most common profile in the population at large, at 14 percent, and with only a relatively slight difference in the male and female populations - respectively 11 percent and 17 percent. Typical characteristics would include the ability to be creative, holistic, and synthesizing in the Upper Right D quadrant, and interpersonal, emotional, and spiritual in the Lower Right C quadrant. The left mode secondaries with logical, analytical, and mathematical thinking styles from Upper Left A, and the organizational, planning, and structure from Lower Left B, would be functional, yet clearly secondary to the preferred right modes of thinking. Those with this profile often have the occupations of teaching or facilitating. Other occupations include the arts, such as writers, musicians, artists, and designers, as well as those in the "helping" fields - psychologists and counselors. This profile could also support entrepreneurial behavior, since it features the imaginative, innovative, and "risk" oriented behavior of the right mode, quadrants C and D, without the control or preference of the structured, logical and conservative modes of the left quadrants A and B.

Herrmann N: The Creative Brain. Lake Lure, NC: Brain Books, 1988. Reprinted with permission by the Ned Herrmann Group.

Appendix C: ALTERNATIVE MUSIC

Composer	Company	Selection	Application
Jon Bernoff & Marcus Allen	Dream Weaver Music BMI/Rising Sun Records	*Breathe.* Environmental sounds mixed with instruments, et al	Side 1: Relaxation Side 2: Up-tempo
Jim Chappell	Unspeakable Freedom Production	*Dusk.* Piano	Contemplation
Rusty Crutcher	Emerald Green Sound Productions	*Machu Picchu Impressions* Environmental & instruments	Associative meditation Yoga exercises
Alex Jones & Doug Cutler	Alex Jones	*Kali's Dream.* Piano	Peacefulness/contemplation
Michael Jones	MCA Records	*Seascapes; After the Rain.*	Peacefulness/contemplation
Kitaro	Polygram	*Silk Road*	Up-tempo; uplifting.
Daniel Kobialka	Lisem	*Timeless Motion; Dream Passage.* Violin, plus. Part of a series.	Relaxation; self-motivation
David Lanz	Narada	*Skyline Firedance; Christofori's Dream.* Piano	Uplifting & relaxing
Ray Lynch	Music West; Windham Hill	*Deep Breakfast; Sky of Mind.* Synthesizers, etc.	DB: up-tempo; uplifting SM: relaxation; meditation
Carlos Nakai	Silver Wave	*Earth Spirit.* Native American flute	Relaxation; meditation
Mike Rowland	Narada	*The Fairy Ring* Piano/synthesizer	Contemplation.
Robert Slap	Valley of the Sun	*Ascension to All That Is* Harp, synthesizer, etc.	Associative and non-associative meditation
Upper Astral	Valley of the Sun	*Crystal Cave: Back to Atlantis.* Harp, synthesized voices	Associative meditation; massage
George Winston	Windham Hill	*December.* Piano	Contemplation

Appendix D: PRINCIPLES OF THE PERENNIAL PHILOSOPHY

The following are extracted primarily from Aldous Huxley's *The Perennial Philosophy* (Ref. #58) and Huston Smith's *The Religions of Man* (Ref. #101). They depict the major esoteric and exoteric traditions found in all principle world religions - from Buddhism, Confucianism, Hinduism through Christianity, Judaism, Islam and Taoism.

1. God *is*. God exists. Attempting to define God is impossible. Attempting to categorize God is impossible. God is within time and exists outside of time. God is within each individual, each creation, yet transcends that creation. God is nothing: ("No-thing") and oneness. God as creator continues to create. God is the continuous, with duality dissolved within the continuous.

2. God can be perceived by humanity, however. Godhead exists or manifests in various aspects, such as Shiva, the Christian trilogy, Jesus, Christ energy, etc.

3. Absolute Godhead is the goal of evolution. God is multidirectional, not unidirectional.God is *not* a one way street for humanity: a permanent descent away from God - a fall from original Grace - into an everlasting state of oritinal sin due to having eaten the forbidden fruit of knowledge. All creation, all that which is created, is to grow back, spiritually return, into Godhead. This is the goal of evolution. This is the meaning for each man and woman. We *shall grow* back into Godhead. This is the meaning of Jesus when he said, "Be in the world but not of the world."

4. Any story of creation is more than a morality play about original sin. The Fall is not so much a fall from grace by all of humanity as a presentation of a person's egocentric free will choosing to create and spin away from God, from Oneness.

5. Each person has free will, choice as to how long the road back will be. The Ground of our Being is Godhead. The within (the Self) wishes to unite with the Without (Godhead).

6. God is in the world *now*. Life is sacred. Humanity's dominion over nature is *not* dominance of nature.

7. God is charity and love. God gives humanity resources for the growth back.

Those range from earth-existence masters (self-realized ones), avatars (Christed ones), guides, guardian angels, presenters, through individual resources: self, ego, mind, brain, body, etc. (Incidentally, Christ was a title bestowed on Jesus, from the Greek, kristos: (CHRISTOS): annointed. Jesus' real title should read, Jesus of Nazareth, the Christed One.) Through the Christ energy in an avatar, God manifests in human form. This hopefully helps explain that most mysterious, mystical New Testament Gospel writer, John.

The more effort a person makes in the attempt at self-knowledge and transcendence of the ego, the more resources are given.

8. God's grace *exists*, encompassing all creation. As the Christian theologian Paul Tillich states, "...[A]ccept the fact that you are accepted!"[1] The gift is a given.

9. Heaven exists within and without. It is timeless. It does not necessarily have to be attained after death. The kingdom of heaven and hell exist within us. It is our choice, given free will.

10. All religions guarantee some type of survival after earth-time existence. What the *quality* will be is determined by each individual.

11. The greater the degree of self awareness, the greater the ability for one to be attached to, yet detached from, ego and earth-related matters. This attainment of self-awareness must be commensurate with mortification of the ego or transcendance of the ego. To transcend the ego, one must develop an ego. To grow out of an ego, one must have an ego.

12. God encompasses and transcends daily. Good *and* evil exist, for example. Heaven *and* hell. Pain and suffering *and* pleasure and happiness. One cannot know and understand one without experiencing *both* it and its opposite.

13. God is love, allowing for growth. Regarding the universe, Einstein stated, God does not throw dice (Ref. #92). There *are* universal laws at work. There *is* order in perceived chaos. Commensurate with the right to grow is the responsibility one *must* shoulder for acts and actions taken and thoughts thought.

In Christianity, one of these is: "What you sow so shall ye reap". Hinduism and Buddhism call it *karma*: the law of cause and effect (positive and negative). By the ancient Greeks, it was called *hubris* and *nemesis:* exaggerated pride and ego leading to retribution. Nature, including human nature, wishes balance and harmony. Imbalance always leads to retribution, in order to restore balance.

14. There are various paths to self-awareness. Each path is meant for a particular personality type for which that path is more natural.

For example, Buddhism encompasses three major ways:

- The Way of Knowledge
- The Way of Works
- The Way of Devotion

From Hinduism, four principal yogas emanate:

- Raja yoga (popular in the west because the popular hatha yoga is a component of raja yoga), the way of psychological exercises
- Jnana yoga, a combination of rationality and spirituality
- Bhakti yoga, the way through love (and devotion). (This also was original Christianity: the love of God through devotion to His only son, Jesus.)
- Karma yoga, the way through works.

---

1 Tillich, P. *The Shaking of the Foundations,* p. 162.

References: 58, 92, 101

Appendix E: IMPLICATIONS OF A TIME-ORIENTED GOD FOR HEALTH AND HEALING

The word *chronological* by definition implies time. A chronological-oriented theology creates a time-oriented God. Such a theology has tremendous implications for the society creating it, including the society's healthcare philosophy and its practice.

The following tenets of such a philosophy and its implications are listed below:

1. The modern health covenant with God: I pray to you, therefore you are to heal me (meaning: physical cure). If you don't, then you are powerless after all; or, I am unworthy of your power (see 6, "original sin", below), if I am not cured.

2. A God is on our side mentality. This leads to entreaties to God to d--n:
    - The other person
    - The other country and its army
    - The other person's religion

3. If I'm good (how **I** define good) in this time-oriented life, I go to heaven.

4. The concept of heaven becomes time-oriented in this theology. How I define heaven in this time-oriented life is how heaven must actually look.

5. A time-oriented God becomes an anthropomorphic God, having human psychological traits and physical characteristics. We thus pray to Him; or, in solemn political correctness, to Her.

6. A time-oriented God is steeped in original sin doctrine. If there is original sin, then I am born guilty and am inherently sinful. This creates a God of punishment and a *quid pro quo* covenant with God (see "1", above).

    This can also lead to a self-fulfilling prophecy: if I am sinful and unworthy, then "what the h---", let's eat, drink, and be merry (or terrorize, rape, steal, and kill - words more appropriate to 20th century America).

7. If God is temporal, then values and ethics associated with God change as that society changes. This leads to:
    - God is dead
    - God is relative, having no place in contemporary (meaning:

time-oriented) society

8. A time-oriented God is a co-dependent god. Co-dependency by its nature implies limits. God is limited.

9. Creation of co-dependent god with limited power creates questions such as:
- Why do bad things happen to good people?
- Why do good things happen to bad people?

10. Creation of a co-dependent god leads to:
- Points 1-9 above
- Worship of other powerful gods, such as: health; money; sex; the devil; etc.

God becomes whatever is the person's ultimate concern - ultimate in the sense of what the person thinks he or she wants, not what he or she needs. Prayer to this god becomes the proverbial wish list.

- A time-oriented culture which includes:
  - The celebrity of the day
  - The fad of the week
  - The fashion of the month

- A time-oriented healthcare system that emphasizes physical cure. Physical cure is the one level of health out of the four listed in Section #5 that is totally time-oriented

A time-oriented culture perpetuating a time-oriented God leads to a time-oriented healthcare system emphasizing physical cure. Point 1 above gives a succinct and practical example of the fallacy involved in the interplay between time-oriented theology and time-oriented healthcare - with its negative consequences.

A time-oriented God and its theology as outlined above is totally contradictory to the principles of the perennial philosophy as outlined in Appendix D.

#31: RESOURCES

The institutions and organizations listed in this section offer training, services, clinical and/or behavioral medicine skills, and/or products to the reader interested in specific areas of patient education and/or mind/body health. (The reader is also encouraged to consult the resources listed in Appendix A and the resources and organizations listed for each chapter of Mind/Body Medicine [Ref. #48]).

The resources listed in this section are composed of three categories:

(1) Healing organizations
(2) Training organizations
(3) Publications and products

1. Healing organizations

AMERICAN CANCER SOCIETY
1599 Clifton Road, NE, Atlanta, GA 30329-4251 (800)ACS-2345
Description: The American Cancer Society is a national community-based health organization offering research and educational services to both the lay person and the healthcare professional. It is dedicated to both treatment and prevention of cancer. Public education emphasizes early detection and primary cancer prevention through nutrition and control of smoking. Professional education emphasizes the best possible techniques of cancer prevention, detection, and management. Through its volunteers and local affiliates, the national organization provides a variety of patient services at the community level. Diverse educational programs and research data are available to the public and the healthcare professional.

AMERICAN PAIN SOCIETY
5700 Old Orchard Road, First Floor, Skokie, IL 60077-1057 (708)966-5595
Description: The American Pain Society is a nonprofit educational and scientific organization whose mission is to serve people by advancing research, education, treatment and professional practice. It is a national network of over 2500 professional members offering world wide access to information on pain treatment. Membership includes information on seminars, workshops, and publications regarding its mission statement. The American Pain Society has published a compact, easily accessible reference guide, "Principles of Analgesic Use in the Treatment of Acute Pain and Cancer Pain", for healthcare professionals.

AMERICAN SELF-HELP CLEARING HOUSE
St. Clares-Riverside Medical Center, 25 Pocono Road, Denville, NJ 07834
(201)625-7101
Description: The center provides people (lay and professional) with contacts for 750 self-help organizations throughout the United States. They will refer individuals to self-help organizations in the inquirer's locale, if such an organization exists. The center also offers technical assistance to callers on how to start support groups. It publishes *The Self-Help Clearing House,* a listing of 750 self-help organizations. This publication is updated every other year.

COMMONWEAL
M. Lerner, PhD, President; R. Naomi Remen, MD, Medical Director, PO Box 316, Bolinas, CA 94924-0316 (415)868-0970
Description: Founded in 1976, Commonweal is a nonprofit health and environmental research institute supported by diverse foundations and public agencies. It offers several programs for both the lay person and the healthcare professional. For example, it offers six-week-long residential workshops each year (at its 60-acre coastal site next to Port Reyes National Seashore) for people with cancer and members of their families or close friends. The goals of this program, the "Commonweal Cancer Help Program", are to:

- Reduce the stress associated with cancer
- Provide mutual support
- Provide choices involving life style behavioral changes & cancer therapies

Several publications related to these goals are available to the public.

THE LEARNING CENTER OF THE UNIVERSITY OF MINNESOTA HOSPITAL AND CLINIC
Contact person: Ms. Nancy L. Goldstein, Coordinator, Patient Education, University of Minnesota Hospital and Clinic, 420 South East Delaware, Minneapolis, MN 55455 (612)626-6356 FAX: (612)626-4102
Description: Refer to Table 10.1, Section #10.

THE MIND/BODY MEDICAL INSTITUTE
Herbert Benson, MD, President, Division of Behavioral Medicine, New England Deaconess Hospital, 185 Pilgrim Rd., Boston, MA 02215 (617)632-9530
Description: The Institute is a nonprofit scientific and educational organization affiliated with the Harvard Medical School and dedicated to the research and application of mind/body behavioral interventions, including the relaxation response, to the field of medicine. It sponsors a variety of professional training programs, including continuing medical education courses in conjunction with

Harvard Medical School, for healthcare professionals. The Institute offers patient-centered workshops such as the "Healthy Life Styles" program, designed for people who recognize that stress is having a negative effect on their life style. Working at the forefront of modern medicine, the Institute serves as a bridge between the traditional separations of mind and body, science and belief, and Eastern and Western medical practice.

PLANETREE HEALTH RESOURCE CENTER
PLANETREE MODEL HOSPITAL UNIT
2300 California St., Suite 201, San Francisco, CA 94115 (415) 923-3680, 923-3681 FAX: (415)673-7650 Walk-in library access: 2040 Webster St., San Francisco, CA 94115
Description: The mission of Planetree, as a nonprofit organization, is to assist organizations in humanizing and demystifying healthcare for patients and their families. These goals are achieved by:

- Providing people with access to health and medical information that will enable them to make informed choices about their healthcare
- Helping healthcare organizations provide humanistic care and create healing patient-centered environments which respond to the needs of the whole person

The Planetree philosophy is to put the ideals and values of humanistic care into the practical realities of healthcare settings in five Model Hospital Sites around the country as examples of patient-centered care.

Planetree also operates the Health Resource Center program. Staff help locate and compile requested medical information. Services are available to both the lay person and the healthcare professional for a modest fee. To receive more information on these services, call (415)923-3681.

PREVENTIVE MEDICINE RESEARCH INSTITUTE
Dean Ornish, MD, President and Director, 900 Bridgeway, Suite 2, Sausalito, CA 94965 (800)328-3738 or (415)332-2525.
Description: Nonprofit organization associated with the School of Medicine, University of California at San Francisco. In addition to conducting ongoing clinical research, it offers training programs in mind/body medicine (such as reducing the effects of atherosclerosis [cardiovascular disease] through diet, meditation, exercise, yoga, and general support groups) for both the healthcare professional and the general public.

STRESS REDUCTION CLINIC
Jon Kabat Zinn, Ph. D., Director, University of Massachusetts Medical Center, Worchester, MA 01655 (508)856-1616
Description: The clinic sponsors the "Stress Reduction and Relaxation Program" at the Medical Center. It is an outpatient behavioral medicine clinic consisting of an eight-week-long course to complement a person's current medical treatment. It is the oldest and largest hospital-based stress reduction clinic in the United States. People must be referred to the clinic by their doctors. Individuals referred have requested treatment for such conditions as:

- Heart disease
- Chronic pain
- Stress and anxiety
- Cancer
- AIDS
- High blood pressure
- Fatigue

Dr. Kabat Zinn's book (Ref. #62) describes the program in detail.

2. Training Organizations

INSTITUTE FOR THE STUDY OF HEALTH AND ILLNESS
Rachel Naomi Remen, MD, Director, COMMONWEAL, PO Box 316, Bolinas, CA 94924-0316 (415)868-2642 FAX: (415)868-2230
Description: The Institute is a professional development institute for health professionals who wish to devote all or part of their practice to serving people with life-threatening illnesses. It offers a series of five residential weekend workshops and optional clinical supervision seminars. One of the Institute's fundamental assumptions is that people cannot function as healers without examining their lives in depth: Who we are has a deep impact on those we work with.

KOMRAS & ASSOCIATES
Henrietta Komras, M.Ed., President, 1515 North Warson, Suite 206, St. Louis, MO 63132 (314)429-5450 FAX:(314)423-1192
Description: Komras & Associates is a consulting firm specializing in both management development and patient focused care training for healthcare personnel. The latter includes training professionals in mind/body behavioral medicine interventions and their application to healing. Provides assistance in the design and development of patient education materials and healing environments within healthcare settings.

MIND/BODY HEALTH SCIENCES, INC.
Joan Borysenko, PhD, President, 393 Dixon Rd., Boulder, CO 80302
(303)440-8460 FAX: (303)440-7580
Description: Publishes a yearly newsletter and accepts requests for lectures, workshops and training by Joan Borysenko, Ph.D., Miron Borysenko, Ph.D., and other prominent professionals. Provides programs for private, community, religious, health, business, and other organizations. Meditations, lectures, workshops, music and other related materials are available on audiotape and may be ordered directly from MBHS, Inc.

THE NED HERRMANN GROUP
Ned Herrmann, President, 2275 Buffalo Creek Rd., Lake Lure, NC 28746
(704)625-9153 FAX: (704)625-2198
Description: Offers training and technical assistance in both administration and analysis of the Herrmann Brain Dominance Instrument (Section #9) and its many applications to both the work environment and one's personal life. Publisher of the International Brain Dominance Review, a quarterly magazine dedicated to brain dominance research and application, and *The Creative Brain* by Ned Herrmann, 440 pages.

RG SWARTZ & ASSOCIATES
RG Swartz, MAEd, MPA, owner, PO Box 7568, Lancaster, PA 17604-7568
(717)299-5061 FAX: (717)560-0522
Description: A consulting organization that: (1) trains trainers in the application of accelerated learning methods to their staff development and patient education programs (Section #10 and Ref. #103); (2) trains healthcare professionals and lay persons to effectively use mind/body healthcare skills in order to promote their own healing; (3) produces books, workbooks, training materials, and audio cassette tapes on these subjects.

3. Publications and products

BRAIN/MIND: A BULLETIN OF BREAKTHROUGHS
Interface Press, Marilyn Ferguson, Publisher, Box 42211, 4717 N. Figueroa St., Los Angeles, CA 90042 (800)553-MIND or (213)223-2500
Description: A publication in newsletter form disseminating synopses of brain/mind research findings from diverse fields, with applications to the healthcare, education, and training fields.

HEALING AND THE MIND WITH BILL MOYERS

Ambrose Video Publishing, 1290 Avenue of the Americas, #2245, New York, NY 10104 Phone: (800)345-2690 (home orders); (800)526-4663 (educational orders) FAX: (212)265-8088

Description: A five-program video cassette series originally presented February 1993 by the Public Broadcasting System (coproduced by: David Brubin Productions, Inc., and Public Affairs Television, Inc.). The series deals with the impact of mind and emotions upon health. Mr. Moyers interviews mind/body researchers as well as healthcare professionals in various settings. Especially poignant are interviews with caregivers using mind/body behavioral medicine skills while experiencing health crises. (One video cassette of this series is alluded to in Section #20.) The Viewer's Guide (developed by: Thirteen/WNET, 356 West 58th St., New York, NY 10019) accompanying the series is designed to provide material for further discussion and experiential material for learning about issues related to the series, as well as a listing of resources related to health and healing.

INTERNATIONAL PATIENT EDUCATION COUNCIL (IPEC)

11512 Allecingie Parkway, Richmond, VA 23235 (804)379-5513

FAX: (804)379-1386

Description: The mission of IPEC is "To advance the science and practice of patient education, in order to promote educationally centered healthcare at the local, regional and international levels." The organization publishes *Patient Education RX* for its members, and the *Journal of Patient Education and Counseling* is published in collaboration with IPEC. Each year, IPEC sponsors National Patient Education Week in the first week of November, and produces a how-to planning packet for the week. An annual conference focuses on issues, trends, networking, and resource sharing.

PATIENT EDUCATION REFERENCE HANDBOOK

Minnesota Chapter, American Society for Healthcare Education and Training, producer. *Contact person*: Nancy Goldstein (See "Learning Center...", under "Healing organizations", above, for address and telephone number.)

Description: Content includes: a patient education resource directory; strategies for increasing patient education visibility within an organization; how to develop patient education materials; training methodology (including video); legal and ethical issues surrounding patient education; quality assurance research; Joint Commission on Accreditation of Healthcare Organizations' standards related to patient education.

References: 48, 62.

#32: REFERENCES

1. Achterberg J: Imagery in healing: Shamanism and modern medicine. Boston: New Science Library, 1985.
2. American Hospital Association: A patient's bill of rights. Chicago, IL, 1980. In: Redman BK: The process of patient education, 7th ed. St. Louis, MO: Mosby-Year Book, Inc., 1993:11-12.
3. Atkinson W: Lighting and office: Cost versus comfort. The Office, 1989; 110:78-80.
4. Bartlett EE: At last, a definition. Patient Education and Counseling, 1985; 7(4):323-324.
5. Bartlett EE: Historical glimpses of patient education in the United States. Patient Education and Counseling, 1986; 8 (nn):135-149
6. Bass MJ, Buck C, Turner L, Dickie G, Pratt G, Campbell RH: The physician's actions and the outcome of illness in family practice. The Journal of Family Practice, 1986; 23(1): 43-47.
7. Begley S: Alternative medicine: A cure for what ails us? American Health 1992; 11(3): 39-46.
8. Benson H. with Klipper MZ: The relaxation response. New York: Avon Books, 1975
9. Benson, H. with Proctor W: Beyond the Relaxation Response. New York: Times Books, 1984.
10. Birren F: Color psychology and color therapy: A factual study of the influence of color on human life. Secaucus, NJ: The Citadel Press, 1961
11. Blendon RJ, Donelan K. Leitman R, Epstein A, Cantor JD, Cohen AB, Morrison I, Moloney T, Koeck C., Levitt SW: Special article: Physicians' perspectives on caring for patients in the United States, Canada, and West Germany. The New England Journal of Medicine 1993: 328 (14): 1011-1016.
12. Blotzer J: Rx: Rationalization: When high-tech medicine is too much of a good thing. Pittsburgh Post Gazette, August 18, 1993; Section B: 2.
13. Borysenko J: Guilt is the Teacher: Love is the lesson. New York: Warner Books, 1990.
14. Borysenko J, with Rothstein L: Minding the body, mending the mind. Reading, MA: Addison-Wesley Publishing Co., Inc., 1987.
15. Breaking the code of musicality. Brain/Mind Bulletin, Special Issue 1985; 10 (4-5):1-8.
16. Burgoon M, Birk TS, Hall Jr: Compliance and satisfaction with physician-patient communications. Human Communication Research 1991: 18(2): 177-208.

17. Burgoon JK, Pfau M, Parrott R, Birk T, Coker, R, Burgoon M: Relational communication, satisfaction, compliance-gaining strategies, and compliance in communication between physicians and patients. Communications Monographs, 1987; 54(2): 307-324.
18. Buzan T: Use both sides of your brain. New York: EP Dutton, 1983.
19. Buzan T: Use your perfect memory. New York: EP Dutton, 1984.
20. Candace Pert: Emotions in body, not just in brain. Brain/Mind Bulletin, 1986; 11(4): 1-2.
21. Caudill M, Schnable R, Zuttermeister P, Benson H, Friedman R: Decreased clinic use by chronic pain patients: Response to behavioral medicine intervention. The Clinical Journal of Pain, 1991; 7(nn): 305-310.
22. Charlesworth EA, Nathan RG: Stress management: A comprehensive guide to wellness, 2nd ed. New York: Ballantine Books, 1984
23. Chopra, D: Quantum healing. New York: Bantam Books, 1989.
24. Clogged arteries, cholesterol levels altered by diet, meditation. Brain/Mind Bulletin, 1988; 14(3), 3.
25. Communication with spouse reduces cardiac risk. Brain/Mind & Common Sense, 1992; 17(12); 1,8.
26. Conlee CJ, Olvera J, Vagim NN: The relationship among physician nonverbal immediacy and measures of patient satisfaction with physician care. Communication Reports, 1993; 6(1):25-33.
27. Cousins N: Head First. New York: Penquin Books, 1989.
28. Cowley G, Hager M, with Leonard EA: Tuberculosis: A deadly return. Newsweek, 1992; 119(11): 52-57.
29. Crane VS: Patient education as a mechanism for illness prevention and self-care. The Health Care Supervisor, 1985; 4(1):58-59.
30. Creditor MC: Hazards of hospitalization of the elderly. Annals of Internal Medicine, 1993; 118(3): 219-223.
31. del Bueno, D: Patient Education: Planning for success. Journal of Nursing Administration, 1978; 8(6):3-7.
32. Devine EC, Cook TD: Clinical and cost-saving effects of psychoeducational interventions with surgical patients. Research in Nursing and Health, 1986; 9(2): 89-105.
33. Devine EC, Cook TD: A meta-analytic analysis of effects of psychoeducational interventions on length of postsurgical hospital stay. Nursing Research, 1983; 32(5): 267-274.
34. Dossey L: Beyond illness: Discovering the experience of health. Boston: New Science Library, 1984.
35. Dossey, L: Recovering the soul. New York: Bantam Books, 1989.

36. Durback E, Nendick P: No frills patient education. Canadian Nurse, 1986; 82(4): 21-23.
37. Eccles, Sir J, Robinson DN: The wonder of being human: Our brain and our mind. Boston: New Science Library, 1985.
38. Eisenberg DM, Kessler RC, Foster C, Norlock FE, Calkins DR, Delbanco TL: Special article: Unconventional medicine in the United States - prevalence, costs, and patterns of use. New England Journal of Medicine, 1993; 328(4): 246-252.
39. Ellis A, Harper RA: A new guide to rational living. N. Hollywood, CA: Wilshire Book Company, 1979.
40. Findlay S, Brownlee S, and Beach L (illus.): The body at war: Baring the secrets of the immune system. US News & World Report, 1991; 111(13): 48-54.
41. Findlay S, Podolsky D, Silberner J: Wonder cures from the fringe. US News & World Report, 1991; 111(13): 68-74.
42. Fox M: Original blessing. Santa Fe, NM: Bear & Company, Inc., 1983.
43. Friedman M, Ulmer D: Treating type A behavior and your heart. New York: Fawcett Crest, 1984.
44. Gagne RM, Briggs W: Principles of Instructional Design. New York: Holt, Reinhart & Winston, 1954.
45. Lick D: New age meets Hippocrates; medicine gets serious about unconventional therapy. Newsweek, 1991; 120(2): 58.
46. Goldstein, NL: Patient learning center: A description of the learning center of the University of Minnesota Hospital and Clinic. Minneapolis, MN, 1993.
47. Goldstein, NL: Patient learning center reduces patient readmissions. Patient Education and Counseling, 1991; 17(nn): 177-190.
48. Goleman D, Gurin J: Mind body medicine: How to use your mind for better health. New York: Consumer Reports paperbacks for better health. New York: Consumer Reports Books, 1993.
49. Grimaldi, PL, Micheletti JA. Diagnosis Related Groups: a practitioner's guide. Chicago, IL; Pluribus Press, Inc., 1983:1-56.
50. Halpern S, Savary L: Sound health; The music and sounds that make us whole. San Francisco: Harper & Row, 1985.
51. Hamlin S: How to talk so people listen. New York: Harper & Row, 1988.
52. Hampden-Turner C: Maps of the mind. New York: Collier Books, 1982.
53. Hay L: You can heal your life; Carson, CA: Hay House, Inc., 1984.
54. Heinz, U.S. Senator John A., Chairman, Special Committee on Aging, US Senate, letter to the Honorable Margaret M. Heckler, Secretary, US Department of Health and Human Services, October 7, 1985, p. 2 in: "Appendix", Quality of care under medicare's prospective payment system: Vol.II (US Government Printing Office: Washington DC), Serial Nos. 98-99, 10, 11, 1986, p. 71.

55. Henry SA, Swartz RG,: Use of accelerated learning techniques in education. The International Brain Dominance Review, 1992; 8(1-2): 6-12.
56. Herrmann N: The creative brain. Lake Lure, NC: Brain Books, 1988.
57. Hurley III TJ: Placebos and healing: A new look at the "Sugar Pill": Institute of Noetic Sciences, 1985; 13(2): 5-8.
58. Huxley A: The perennial philosophy. New York: Harper & Row, 1945, 1990.
59. Jacubowski P, Lange AJ: The assertive option: Your rights and responsibilities. Chicago, IL: Research Press Company, 1978.
60. Janiger O, Goldberg P: A different kind of healing: Doctors speak candidly about their successes with alternative medicine. New York: GP Putnam's Sons, 1993.
61. Joint Commission on Accreditation of Healthcare Organizations: Section I: Education of patients and family.1996 Comprehensive Accreditation Manual for Hospitals: Volume I Standards. Oak Brook Terrace, IL,1996; 209-210.
62: Kabat-Zinn J: Full catastrophe living: Using the wisdom of body and mind to face stress, pain, and illness. New York: Dell Publishing, 1990.
63. Knowles M: The adult learner: A neglected species, 2nd ed. Houston: Gulf Publishing Co., 1978.
64. Lange AJ, Jacobowski P with McGovern TV: Responsible assertive behavior: Cognitive/behavioral procedures for trainers. Champaign, IL: Research Press, 1976.
65. Long HB: Adult learning: Research and practice. Cambridge: Cambridge Book Co.,1983; 38-70.
66. Leading researcher challenges 'genetic paradigm'. Brain/Mind & Common Sense, 1993; 18(9): 1, 6.
67. Leaf A: Special communication: Preventive medicine for our ailing health care system. Journal of the American Medical Association, 1993; 269(5): 616-618.
68. Lipetz MJ, Bussigel MN, Bannerman J, Risley B: What is wrong with patient education programs? Nursing Outlook, 1990; 38(4): 184-189.
69. Mager R: Preparing Instructional Objectives, 2nd ed. Belmont, CA: Fearon-Pitman Publishers, Inc., 1975.
70. Magill K, Caspi A: Patient education; Progress and problems. Nursing Management 1986; 17(2): 44-49.
71. Margen S and the editors of the University of California at Berkeley Wellness Letter: The wellness encyclopedia of food and nutrition. New York: Rebus/ Random House, 1992, pp.11-38.
72. Meer J: The light touch. Psychology Today, 1985; 19(9): 60-67.
73. 'Mind-gene connection' links disease and learning. Brain/Mind Bulletin, 1986; 11(16): 1-2.

74. Moyers B: The art of healing. A videocassette of the series: Healing and the mind - with Bill Moyers. New York. Ambrose Video Publishing, 1993.
75. Multiple personality no longer considered rare. Brain/Mind Bulletin, 1988; 14(2): 1-2.
76. Mumford E, Schlesinger HJ, Glass GV: The effects of psychological intervention on recovery from surgery and heart attacks: An analysis of the literature. American Journal of Public Health, 1982; 72(2): 141-151.
77. Mutual of Omaha set to pay for preventive care in pilot program. Brain/Mind Bulletin of Breakthroughs 1993; 18(10): 1,6.
78. Narrow B: Patient teaching in nursing practice. New York: John Wiley & Sons, 1979.
79. O'Regan B: Healing, remission and miracle cures. Institute of Noetic Sciences Special Report, 1987; 5(nn): 1-14.;
80. Olga M, Finnen RT, Minor-Schork D, and Payne G: Go for the gold - RN: A support program for graduate nurses. Perspectives on Patient Care (Greenville. NC: Pitt County Memorial Hospital), 1990; 4(2): 5-8.
81. Ornstein R, Sobel D: The healing brain: Breakthrough discoveries about how the brain keeps us healthy. New York: Simon and Schuster, 1987.
82. Ornstein R, Sobel D: Healthy pleasures. Reading, MA: Addison-Wesley, 1989.
83. Ornstein R, Thompson RF, Macaulay D (illus): The amazing brain. Boston: Houghton Mifflin, 1984.
84. Ostrander S, Schroeder L, Ostrander N: Superlearning. New York: Dell Publishing, 1979.
85. Patient education injects quality into health care. International Patient Education Council Resource Sheet 1989; 1-4.
86. Pelletier KR: Mind as healer, mind as slayer: A holistic approach to preventing stress disorders. New York: Dell Publishing, 1977.
87. Peptides: population explosion in brain chemicals. Brain Mind Bulletin, 1984; 9(5); 3.
88. Pike A, McHugh M, Canney K, Miller N., Reiley P., Seibert C: A new architecture for quality assurance. Journal of Nursing Care quarterly, 1993; 7(3): 1-8.
89. Podolsky D: Fringe medicine: Big claims, no proof. US News & World Report, 1991; 111(13): 77
90. Postlethwait S: An integrated experience approach in learning. Minneapolis, MN: Burgess Publishing Co., 1964.
91. Postlethwait, S: Minicourse: Focusing on the individual and his learning. The Library College Journal, 1971: 4(1): 16:23.

92. Prigogine I, Stengers I with Toffler A: Order Out of Chaos: Man's new dialogue with nature. Boulder, CO: New Science Library/Shambhala Publications Inc., 1984.
93. Redman BK: The process of patient education, 7th ed., St. Louis, MO: Mosby-Year Book, Inc. 1993.
94. Religious faith, mental health linked by "hard" data. New Sense Bulletin, 1992; 17(5); 1, 8.
95. Remen N: Healing and wholeness: Living well and dying well. Institute of Noetic Sciences, 1986; 14(1): 3-7.
96. Roter DL, Hall JA: Doctors talking with patients/patients talking with doctors: Improving communication in medical visits. Patients talking with doctors. Improving communication in medical visits. Westport,CT: Auburn House, 1992.
97. Rubin R, Zimmerman R (illus.): Cholesterol, Round 2. US News & World Report, 1993; 114(25): 61-66.
98. Seyle H: Stress without distress. New York: Harper & Row, 1974.
99. Siegel, BS: Love, medicine & miracles. New York: Harper & Row, 1986.
100. Simonton OC, Matthews-Simonton S, Creighton JL: Getting well again. New York: Bantam Books, 1978.
101. Smith H: The religions of man. New York: Harper & Row, 1958.
102. Success with multiples called 'hope of the 80's'. Brain/Mind Bulletin, 1985; 11(3): 1-2.
103. Swartz RG: Accelerated learning: how you learn determines what you learn. Durant, OK: Essential Medical Information Systems, Inc., 1991.
104. Tame D: The secret power of music. New York: Destiny Books, 1984.
105. Tieney D, Eisenberg MG: Evaluating patient health education printed materials. Hospital Topics, 1986; 64(2): 28-29, 33.
106. Tillich P: The shaking of the foundations. New York: Charles Scribner's Sons, 1948, 1978.
107. Two-way communication links brain, white cells. Brain/Mind Bulletin, 1988; 14(3): 1.
108. Tyner R: Office lighting and affect your profits. The Office, 1986; 103: 113-114.
109. Wallis C: Why new age medicine is catching on. Time, 1991; 138(18): 68-75.
110. Wilbur K: Eye to eye: The quest for the new paradigm. Boston, MA: Shambhala Publications, Inc., 1990.
111. Williamson KC, McCray N: Putting together a patient education program that works. RN, 1977; 40(11): 53-55.
112. Winson J: Brain & psyche: The biology of the unconscious. New York: Vintage Books, 1985.

113. Woolley FR, Kane RL, Hughes CC, Wright DD: The effects of doctor-patient communication on satisfaction and outcome of care. Social Science and Medicine, 1978; 12(nn): 123-128.
114. Zweig C: Mind and healing. Institute of Noetic Sciences Newsletter. Winter 1985-86; 13(3): 9-11.

Biographical Notes

Gretchen Peske, R.N., M.S.N.

Gretchen Peske, R.N., M.S.N., is owner and Executive Director of the Pulmonary Therapy Group. Located in Greensburg, PA, this free-standing out-patient facility is committed to increasing the health and well-being of people with lung diseases through diagnostics and therapeutic rehabilitation. As author of "Be In Control of Your Lungs", Mrs. Peske enthusiastically teaches the pulmonary patients how to achieve a maximal level of functioning in their daily lives.

Professionally, the setting in which she works offers the roles of clinician, educator and researcher. A graduate of Barry University and Edinboro University of Pennsylvania, she is active in the national organizations of: AACVPR (American Association of Cardiovascular and Pulmonary Rehabilition), ATS (American Thoracic Society), ANA (American Nurses Association), ant Sigma Theta Tau International Nursing Honor Society.

Roger G. Swartz, M.A. Ed., M.P.A.

Roger Swartz, M.A.Ed., M.P.A., is owner of R.G.Swartz & Associates. Located in Lancaster, PA, this consultancy organization specializes in the application of accelerated learning and mind/body behavioral intervention skills to one's professional development and personal growth.

Mr. Swartz is author of *Accelerated Learning: **How** You Learn Determines **What** You Learn* (Essential Medical Information Systems, Inc., 1991). This book received national acclaim in the *Training and Development Journal* of the American Society for Training and Development (May, 1992); and in the winter newsletter of the American Society for Healthcare Education and Training (January, 1993). His workbook, "Music to Learn By", and audiocassette tape, "Sound Learning", received international acclaim in the *Training and Development Journal*, published by the United Kingdom's Institute for Training and Development (November, 1992). Mr. Swartz holds an A.B. degree from Albright College, Reading, PA (1967); and Master degrees from Lehigh University (M.A.Ed., 1969; M.P.A., 1981).

He is also an American Revolutionary war historian. His book, *Frankstown: Anatomy of an Ambush* (Blue Path Press, 1995), received national acclaim in *Muzzleloader* magazine (Nov./Dec., 1995).

Karen Pennebaker, B.A.

Karen Pennebaker graduated from Penn State with a B.A. degree in The Arts, in the School of Art and Architecture, majoring in art. She has been typing/word processing/computing, in that order, for over 35 years. Mrs. Pennebaker designed this book's cover, formatted the book, doing both the typesetting and the layout, as well as some of the illustrations. An award-winning artist, her paintings, hand printed block prints, jewelry and dreamcatchers are in collections all over the world. She conducts workshops for elementary school children in art, especially in block printing, and in publishing and illustrating.